Diagnosis and Management of
Acute Poisoning

Diagnosis and Management is a series of textbooks covering the major fields of medicine and the sub-specialties. The emphasis throughout is placed primarily on providing practical guidance for the clinician with a diagnostic or management problem. The books will also be of value to candidates preparing for a higher degree, general practitioners and senior medical students.

Although some may not consider acute poisoning to be a specialty in its own right, the management of the poisoned comprises a major component of the in-patient workload in many medical units. The number of episodes of acute poisoning continue to increase and the agents available for poisoning proliferate. This textbook first discusses the general principles of diagnosis and management and then deals in detail with specific agents. The alphabetical arrangement ensures easy referral and the text is augmented with numerous references. Based on Dr A. T. Proudfoot's extensive practical knowledge, this volume provides a concise, authoritative and up-to-date guidance for the clinician.

J. F. MUNRO
Series Editor

Diagnosis and Management of Acute Poisoning

ALEXANDER T. PROUDFOOT
BSc MB ChB FRCPE
Consultant Physician,
Regional Poisoning Treatment Centre,
Royal Infirmary, Edinburgh.
Director,
Scottish Poisons Information Bureau

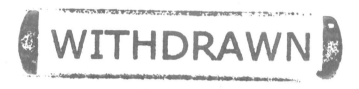
BLACKWELL SCIENTIFIC PUBLICATIONS
OXFORD   LONDON   EDINBURGH
BOSTON   MELBOURNE

© 1982 by
Blackwell Scientific Publications
Editorial offices:
Osney Mead, Oxford, OX2 0EL
8 John Street, London, WC1N 2ES
9 Forrest Road, Edinburgh, EH1 2QH
52 Beacon Street, Boston
     Massachusetts 02108, USA
99 Barry Street, Carlton,
     Victoria 3052, Australia

First published 1982

Typeset by CCC,
printed and bound in Great Britain
by William Clowes (Beccles) Limited,
Beccles and London

DISTRIBUTORS

USA
Blackwell Mosby Book Distributors
11830 Westline Industrial Drive
St. Louis, Missouri 63141

Canada
Blackwell Mosby Book Distributors
120 Melford Drive, Scarborough
Ontario, M1B 2X4

Australia
Blackwell Scientific Book Distributors
214 Berkeley Street, Carlton
Victoria 3053

British Library
Cataloguing in Publication Data

Proudfoot, Alexander T.
    Diagnosis and management of
    acute poisoning.
    1. Poisoning
    I. Title
    615.9   RA1211

    ISBN 0–632–00584–X

Contents

Preface

Acute poisoning is, and is likely to remain, one of the most common medical emergencies. Responsibility for its immediate management, often at unsocial hours, continues to fall on casualty officers and junior physicians, and it is at them that this book is principally directed. Hopefully senior medical students and postgraduates will also find it useful.

Although the book is essentially a practical guide, and therefore fairly dogmatic, I hope it will stimulate some readers to adopt a more thoughtful approach to the diagnosis and management of poisoning than is currently prevalent. For this reason I have tried to indicate uncertainty or lack of knowledge where relevant and have given a limited number of references to original articles on each poison. Papers on poisoning tend to be scattered widely, often in obscure journals, and though the references listed in this book are not always the most important, they are recent and provide an entry to the earlier literature. The considerable advances made in methods of drug analysis in recent years have provoked a much more critical approach to clinical toxicology than was previously possible. Those tempted to contribute to the literature on poisoning should appreciate the importance of confirmatory laboratory evidence for their observations.

Over the years I have had the great good fortune of working closely first with Dr Henry Matthew, then with Dr L. F. Prescott both of whom have made outstanding contributions to clinical toxicology. I and this book owe a great deal to their teaching and example. I am particularly grateful to Drs L. F. Prescott, J. F. Munro, R. N. Illingworth, J. A. J. H. Critchley and R. H. Robson who read and advised on the manuscript. Their comments were generous, sometimes humorous, occasionally contradictory but always constructive.

My special thanks go to Mrs Sheena Turpie who typed the manuscript from impossibly bad handwriting, Mrs Ann Orr who searched the literature indexes and obtained appropriate reprints and Mrs Mamie Strathdee who has helped in innumerable ways.

ATP August 1981

CHAPTER 1

Classification of poisoning

Poisoning episodes may be classified into four types, of which only two are common.

ACCIDENTAL POISONING

Accidental poisoning is most frequently encountered in children between the ages of 1 and 5 years and is the usual cause of poisoning in this age group. At this age it is the consequence of newly-acquired independent mobility, innate curiosity and a predilection for exploring the environment with the mouth as well as the eyes and fingers. It is commonly held that adults facilitate this form of poisoning by leaving household cleaning agents, toiletries and drugs within easy reach in cupboards, beneath kitchen sinks, on bedside tables and in unlocked bathroom cabinets. However, recent studies have shown that accidental poisoning in childhood is not simply a matter of overactivity and ready accessibility of poisons. Homes in which a child poisoning occurs are no more dangerous in terms of availability of potential poisons but are much more likely to have been disturbed by a recent house removal, pregnancy, physical or mental illness in one of the parents or by one parent being away from home. These events may predispose to poisoning episodes by reducing supervision and increasing the availability of drugs.

Accidental poisoning may occur in older children and adults particularly as a result of mishaps at school or work, e.g. inhalation of gases such as chlorine or fumes from organic solvents, ingestion of chemical reagents while pipetting, or drinking some toxic fluid which has been decanted into a soft-drink or beer bottle.

Accidental poisoning with drugs may also occur in confused elderly patients prescribed large numbers of medicines. They may forget the dose and frequency with which each should be taken and make mistakes. While the underlying problem may be arteriosclerotic dementia, confusion and forgetfulness are frequently aggravated or precipitated by inappropriate psychotropic medications.

DELIBERATE SELF-POISONING

Deliberate self-poisoning is the commonest form of poisoning in adults and accounts for at least 95 per cent of all poisoning admissions to hospital. It is sometimes referred to as attempted suicide, parasuicide or pseudocide. This form of poisoning is more common in women. Such patients intentionally take poisons or overdoses of drugs, often impulsively, after a disagreement with a key person in their lives. At the moment of crisis little or no thought is given to the risk, and the possible outcome is of no immediate concern. Most patients, however, have no wish to die. They soon regret their actions and willingly seek medical help. A minority of adults who poison themselves are intent on dying and carefully plan the event, ascertaining as far as possible the toxicity and likely fatal dose of a drug, accumulating a sufficient quantity and taking it under circumstances which make intervention by others improbable. These patients are usually profoundly depressed or psychotic. Another small group of adults deliberately take poisons to teach others a lesson or to manipulate them into an attitude or course of action that they would otherwise reject.

The peak age incidence for self-poisoning is between the ages of 20 and 35 years, but it is not uncommon before the age of 15 years. Self-poisoning should be suspected in any episode occurring over the age of 8 years.

HOMICIDAL POISONING

Acute poisoning as a method of homicide is very uncommon. Sporadic cases occur but in most the poisoning is subacute or chronic as with antimony, arsenic and thallium. In recent years paraquat and ricin have been used as single dose homicidal poisons causing an acute illness.

NON-ACCIDENTAL POISONING

Non-accidental poisoning is the term given to the deliberate administration of a poison to a child by one of its parents and may be regarded as an extension of the battered-child syndrome. It may be more common than is generally appreciated. The causes are not clear, but there is usually disharmony between the parents and the child's illness may be used by one parent to distress the other or to help reduce marital tension by making the child the focus of attention.

Although most poisoning episodes can be readily allocated to one of these categories, occasionally this may be difficult. This is particularly the case when trying to decide whether mild intoxication in elderly patients has been the result of confusion and therapeutic misadventure or deliberate self-poisoning. Similarly overdosage in drug addicts is often regarded as accidental but could equally be classified as self-poisoning. The latter view is recommended.

POINTS OF EMPHASIS

- Accidental poisoning is most frequent between the ages of 1 and 5 years.
- Self-poisoning should be considered in any episode over the age of 8 years but the peak incidence is between 20 and 35 years.
- Most adults who poison themselves act impulsively and have no wish to die.
- Homicidal poisoning is rare but non-accidental poisoning in children may be more common than is generally appreciated.

CHAPTER 2

Diagnosis of poisoning

In the great majority of cases, a diagnosis of acute poisoning is reached on the history given by the patient, by a witness to the episode or on circumstantial evidence. The findings on physical examination may help corroborate the nature of the suspected poison but, in isolation, are seldom sufficiently characteristic to make an unassailable diagnosis of poisoning. The diagnosis can, of course, be made in the absence of any history, circumstantial evidence or typical physical signs by finding high plasma concentrations of drugs, though reliable laboratory screening services are available in only a few centres.

HISTORY

Adults

About 80 per cent of adults who take poisons are conscious on arrival at hospital, and it is not usually difficult to elicit a history of self-poisoning.

Nature of the poison

The patients' statements about the nature of the poisons ingested should be accepted with caution since the drugs found on analysis of blood or urine often correlate poorly with those alleged to have been taken. As a result, some clinicians believe that patients are at best completely unreliable or at worst deliberately misleading. Undoubtedly some do lie about the nature of the drug or poison taken, but the majority are probably as truthful as their knowledge permits. Many patients do not know what they have taken, because they took the first tablets that came to hand and in about 15 per cent of cases these have been prescribed for some other person. Incredibly, others blindly take un-named drugs bought or offered free in public houses in the expectation they they will make them 'feel good'. Intoxication with alcohol at the time of self-poisoning is a common reason for ignorance of the poison taken. To some extent the nature of the drug may be corroborated by descriptions of the tablets or capsules, identification of remaining pills or from labels on containers. While an element of scepticism about patients' statements is clinically healthy there is often no choice but to accept them since it would be impracticable, expensive and unnecessary to obtain laboratory confirmation in every case.

Quantity of the poison

Statements about the quantity of poison taken are even more open to question. A minority of individuals deliberately exaggerate or understate the quantity they have taken according to whether they wish to attract attention or play-down the episode. Most, however, are uncertain about quantities simply because they do not count the number of tablets but take them by the handful not knowing how many were in the bottle in the first place. Again uncertainty about quantity is often due to the influence of alcohol.

Unconscious patients

When adults are found unconscious and a history is not available, a diagnosis of poisoning involves the exclusion of other causes of coma (p. 16) and consideration of circumstantial evidence. The possibility of poisoning must never be dismissed because of the protestations of relatives that the patient would never take an overdose or that no drugs were available. Close relatives are often the last to recognise emotional distress in other members of the household. It must be remembered that drug overdosage is one of the commonest causes of coma in young and middle-aged adults.

Drug overdosage is virtually certain if individuals are found unconscious with empty tablet bottles or a few tablets scattered nearby. When gas is used, the patient may have tried to seal off doors and windows. Suicide notes often make their actions and intentions clear. On other occasions patients may go to unusual places or to remote countryside to take overdoses and may deliberately divest themselves of objects that might identify them should they be discovered. The absence of such identifying articles should raise the suspicion of poisoning.

Children

Accidental poisoning in children is usually a matter of conjecture. A toddler may be found with an open container and/or with hands, face, clothing and surrounding floor soiled with some household product or disintegrated tablets. Under these circumstances it is reasonable to assume that some may have been ingested. In other cases an older child may report that a poison has been taken. In the absence of a witness to the act of poisoning the diagnosis may be suspected from abnormal behaviour, convulsions, ataxia or gastro-intestinal disturbances.

Deliberate poisoning of others

Homicidal poisoning and non-accidental poisoning may be extremely difficult to recognise and require a high index of suspicion. Adults may express the fear that they are being poisoned but young children cannot. In the latter inexplicable features, particularly convulsions, drowsiness and staggering occurring in an episodic manner, should arouse suspicion. Complete recovery usually occurs after removal from the home environment but symptoms may recur after discharge or even while in hospital. In the latter case they can be related to a parental visit. Careful questioning may reveal suspicious deaths or illness in siblings, availability of drugs to parents and psychological stresses in the family. A history of self-poisoning or drug misuse in the parents is not unusual.

SYMPTOMS AND SIGNS

In most cases of poisoning the patients are able to tell what has been taken and symptoms are of relatively little diagnostic value. However, their presence or absence may give some indication of the severity. Many poisons affect multiple body systems and symptoms are frequently numerous and non-specific. Similarly, physical signs appear in clusters rather than singly and are of particular importance in establishing a diagnosis in unconscious patients.

Alimentary features

Pain and ulceration of the oral cavity

Pain and ulceration of the mouth, throat and tongue follow the ingestion of strong alkalis or acids. Among the most common are solutions of paraquat, phenols and sodium hydroxide. Clinitest tablets may become adherent to the buccal and oesophageal mucosa and cause burns by virtue of their sodium hydroxide content. Domestic bleaches are also alkaline but are not sufficiently strong to produce much mucosal damage or mouth pain. Strong acids produce similar symptoms, but though phenols and cresols (as in Lysol) cause buccal burns they are generally painless because of destruction of pain fibres. The burns may not be obvious for 24–36 hours.

Salivation

Increased salivation is occasionally seen in patients who have taken large quantities of chlormethiazole, phencyclidine, cholinesterase inhibitors (organophosphate and carbamate insecticides) and inorganic iodides and bromides. The last named may also cause enlargement of the salivary glands.

Dry mouth

Dryness of the tongue and mouth is often due to anticholinergic compounds but must be interpreted with caution in the presence of mouth breathing and hyperventilation.

Nausea and vomiting

Nausea and vomiting are probably the most common non-specific alimentary symptoms of poisoning. They may be due to direct irritation of the gastric mucosa or to a central effect after absorption of some drugs including narcotics and digoxin. In such cases nausea and vomiting usually comes on within a few hours. If the onset is delayed for 24–36 hours other causes such as hepatic necrosis, pancreatitis or renal failure may be responsible.

Abdominal pain and diarrhoea

Generalised abdominal pain and diarrhoea starting shortly after ingestion are usually due to corrosives which irritate the gastrointestinal tract, e.g. laxatives, strong alkalis and acids, iron salts, colchicine or mercuric chloride. Pain which is delayed in onset is often more localised, right-subcostal discomfort usually being due to hepatic damage and bilateral loin or renal angle pain to renal tubular necrosis.

Loss of bowel sounds

Reduction of bowel sounds often occurs in patients who are deeply unconscious but abdominal distension and ileus are rare. Narcotics and anticholinergic compounds are particularly likely to abolish bowel sounds but activity returns rapidly as consciousness is regained.

Jaundice

Hepatocellular jaundice due to poisons takes 2–3 days to develop and is, therefore, of little diagnostic value since most patients are admitted within 24 hours of the poisoning. Paracetamol is by far the most commonly encountered hepatotoxin. Carbon tetrachloride, other halogenated hydrocarbons, phenylbutazone and the death-cap mushroom, *Amanita phalloides*, should also be considered. Less commonly, jaundice may be due to haemolysis by chlorate, nomifensine or arsine.

Cerebral and neuromuscular features

Staggering and dizziness

Overdoses of central nervous system depressants cause staggering, dizziness, stiffness and weakness. These symptoms are the result of neuromuscular incoordination which can be confirmed by demonstrating nystagmus or carrying out the finger–nose test.

Coma

Coma is one of the most common signs of poisoning and is usually due to direct CNS depression by hypnotics, antidepressants, other anticholinergic drugs, anticonvulsants, tranquillisers, narcotic analgesics (opiates), alcohols and glycols. It is an uncommon feature of severe salicylate poisoning and does not occur with paracetamol intoxication unless another drug, such as dextropropoxyphene (as in Distalgesic), has been taken simultaneously, or hepatic encephalopathy has developed. Many hydrocarbons are volatile and lipid-soluble and may cause coma when ingested (e.g. trichlorethane, trichlorethylene and other dry-cleaning and degreasing agents) or inhaled (as with most substances 'sniffed' by solvent abusers). Coma may also be caused indirectly by hypoglycaemia following administration of insulin and sulphonylureas.

Reflex changes

Hypotonia and hyporeflexia are usual with overdosage of barbiturates, most other hypnotics and phenothiazines. Hypertonia, hyperreflexia and myoclonus are commonly due to poisoning with anticholinergic compounds, sympathomimetic drugs and monoamine oxidase inhibitors.

Anticholinergic compounds also cause extensor plantar reflexes but with deepening coma muscle tone decreases and limb and plantar reflexes may only be elicited with difficulty.

Convulsions

Convulsions may be produced indirectly by hypoglycaemia and hypoxia but are more commonly due to CNS stimulation by a wide variety of chemicals, including anticholinergic compounds, sympathomimetic drugs, monoamine oxidase inhibitors, narcotic analgesics, mefenamic acid and rarely salicylates, cycloserine, camphor, isoniazid and gamma-benzene hexachloride. Patients poisoned with these substances frequently show other signs of heightened neuromuscular excitability (see above). Loud noises and painful stimuli may be sufficient to trigger convulsions.

Dystonic reactions

Dystonic reactions involving the mouth, eyes and head may be caused by metoclopramide, haloperidol, trifluperazine and prochlorperazine.

Delirium and hallucinations

Anticholinergic compounds, sympathomimetics, LSD, phencyclidine, and some mushrooms may cause delirium and hallucinations. These features are more often seen in patients recovering from the anticholinergic syndrome (p. 64) than in the early stages of poisoning. Occasionally they may be due to acute withdrawal of hypnotics or alcohol (delirium tremens).

Ocular features

Blurring of vision

Many patients complain of blurring of vision or inability to focus after overdoses of psychotropic drugs and in most they are due to generalised CNS depression. When anticholinergic drugs have been taken, difficulty in focussing is the result of paralysis of accommodation.

Loss of vision

Partial or complete loss of vision is most likely to be due to quinine or methanol.

Pupil changes

Ocular signs are common and while they are valuable diagnostic features, too much importance has been attributed in the past to pupil size and reactions. It is equally important to appreciate that other signs, such as unequal pupils and divergence of the optic axes, also occur in poisoning and are not necessarily evidence of brain damage or raised intracranial pressure.

Very small or pin-point pupils (particularly in conjunction with a reduced respiratory rate) suggest opiate or cholinesterase inhibitor poisoning while dilated pupils are most commonly due to overdosage of drugs with anticholinergic actions (tricyclic antidepressants, antihistamines, orphenadrine, benztropine, glutethimide and thioridazine). Dilated pupils may also be seen in intoxication with LSD and sympathomimetic drugs including amphetamines, other appetite suppressants, ephedrine and theophylline and its derivatives.

Not uncommonly, the pupils may be unequal in size while the patient is unconscious and become equal as consciousness is regained. There is no explanation for this phenomenon but its occurrence, particularly in isolation, is not a sign of rising intracranial pressure nor an indication for urgent neurosurgery.

Strabismus

Divergent strabismus is frequently found in unconscious poisoned patients. Divergence of the optical axes occurs normally during sleep and may affect the vertical as well as the horizontal axis. It was present at some stage in 42 per cent of 219 consecutive admissions with tricyclic antidepressant poisoning. The incidence following overdosage with hypnotic drugs has not been studied but is undoubtedly common.

Papilloedema

Papilloedema is uncommon in acute poisoning and is usually due to cerebral oedema secondary to prolonged hypoxia. Carbon monoxide, methanol and glutethimide are the only poisons known to be regularly associated with papilloedema.

Nystagmus

Nystagmus is only seen in acute poisoning when the patient is sufficiently conscious to make ocular movements. It is a valuable sign of continuing intoxication and may be present when dysarthria and ataxia have largely disappeared. The nystagmus is usually rapid, fine and best detected on lateral gaze but in more intoxicated patients it may be rotatory, coarse and present on the slightest eye movement. Most commonly it is found during recovery from poisoning with psychotropic drugs but may also be due to phenytoin intoxication.

Subconjunctival haemorrhage

Subconjunctival haemorrhage, often extensive, may be found in young patients, especially girls. It is partly the result of raised venous pressure, particularly during vomiting and difficult gastric lavage, and partly due to the effects of salicylates on platelets and capillaries. Though there may be associated facial purpura it is uncommon to find retinal haemorrhages.

Respiratory features

Cough, sputum production, wheeze and breathlessness

Cough, sputum production, wheeze and breathlessness often occur after inhalation of irritant gases such as ammonia, chlorine, smoke from fires and the oxides of nitrogen but are more likely to be due to pre-existing chronic obstructive airways disease or an aspiration pneumonia.

Cyanosis

Cyanosis in the unconscious patient is usually due to a combination of various factors including respiratory obstruction, hypoxaemia secondary to hypoventilation and ventilation-perfusion imbalance, peripheral vasoconstriction, hypotension and hypothermia. In most cases cyanosis can be abolished by attention to the airway, increasing the oxygen content of the inspired air or by assisted ventilation. Failure of these measures should suggest the possibility that the cyanosis is due to methaemoglobinaemia caused by poisons such as chlorates, phenol, paraquat and aniline.

Hypoventilation

Hypoventilation is common with serious overdosage with any CNS depressant and usually involves the depth of respiration.

Marked reduction in respiratory rate is much less common and is usually due to opiate intoxication.

Hyperventilation

Hyperventilation in the absence of a cardiac or respiratory cause or metabolic acidosis is most commonly due to salicylate overdosage and occasionally to CNS stimulant drugs, cyanide or phenoxyacetic acid herbicides.

Non-cardiac pulmonary oedema

Non-cardiac pulmonary oedema may be caused by a variety of poisons though the mechanisms are not fully understood. Inhaled poisons (e.g. chlorine, ammonia and the oxides of nitrogen) damage the respiratory epithelium directly as does paraquat taken orally.

Pulmonary oedema due to narcotic analgesics and ethchlorvynol (commonly seen in addicts) or salicylates is thought to be due to disruption of pulmonary capillary integrity.

Cardiovascular features

Loss of pulses

Loss of pulses due to peripheral circulatory failure may occur in overdosage with CNS depressants and beta-adrenergic blockers. Rarely, it may be the result of intense arterial constriction caused by ergotamine.

Tachycardia and bradycardia

Tachycardia may be due to poisoning with anticholinergic compounds, sympathomimetic drugs and salicylates while bradycardia (other than that due to hypothermia) may be caused by cardiac glycosides, beta-adrenergic blockers and cholinesterase inhibitors (carbamate and organophosphate insecticides).

Dysrhythmias

Dysrhythmias may be caused by a variety of drugs including cardiac glycosides, anticholinergic compounds (particularly the tricyclic antidepressants), sympathomimetics, phenothiazines, chloral hydrate and antimalarials.

Hypotension

Hypotension may occur in any severe poisoning. Central nervous system depressants commonly lower the systolic blood pressure to about 70–90 mmHg, the extent of the fall being greater with increasing depth of coma. Anticholinergic drugs are less likely to produce severe hypotension than barbiturates. These drugs and other poisons (e.g. paraquat, beta-blockers, antimalarials and iron salts) in massive doses produce hypotension by depressing myocardial contractility. Others do so by reducing the circulating blood volume through gastrointestinal loss of fluid (iron salts, mercuric chloride, strong acids and alkalis, colchicine, paraquat) or by causing venous pooling. Diuretics in overdosage produce hypotension by depleting the intravascular volume and other hypotensive drugs (bethanidine, debrisoquine and guanethidine) by their effect on postganglionic adrenergic nerve fibres. It must also be remembered that severe bradycardia or tachycardia may be associated with hypotension.

Hypertension

Hypertension is uncommon in acute poisoning but may be caused by sympathomimetic drugs, phencyclidine and monoamine oxidase inhibitors. Rarely, overdosage with clonidine results in hypertension rather than hypotension.

Skin

Previous self-injury

Careful examination of the skin, notably the flexor aspects of the wrists and forearms, may yield useful evidence of previous self-injury. Scars in other areas, especially face and neck, may also have been self-inflicted while those on the chest and abdomen are more likely to have been inflicted by another party.

Evidence of addiction

Particular attention must be paid to the skin of the arms, hands and feet. Venepuncture marks, abscesses, ulcers and thrombophlebitis usually indicate that the patient is a drug addict who has recently been mainlining. These findings should alert the medical and nursing staff to the potential risk of serum hepatitis and appropriate protective measures should be taken when handling the patient, or his blood and excreta. Unconscious addicts are likely to be poisoned with opiates or barbiturates, with or without ethanol.

Extensive bruising

Extensive bruising of the head, face, arms and legs suggests physical violence or the possibility of falls following intoxication with ethanol or drugs. Their presence makes it particularly important to consider skull fractures and subdural haematoma.

Purpura

Purpura, like subconjunctival haemorrhage, occurs frequently after emesis or struggling during gastric lavage. It is usually confined to the eyelids but may occasionally spread to the rest of the face and neck. Raised venous pressure, with or without the effects of aspirin, is usually the cause. Rarely it may be seen in young patients after protracted paroxysms of coughing following inhalation of respiratory tract irritants such as chlorine and the oxides of nitrogen. It is important to appreciate the benign nature of this form of purpura so that patients and parents can be reassured that it will disappear in a few days and to prevent unnecessary haematological investigation.

Blistering

Patients who have lain unconscious in the same position for many hours may have erythematous areas of skin over bony prominences and pressure areas when they are found. Within a few hours of the pressure being relieved the lesions may extend in size, become raised with a *peau d'orange* appearance, and go on to blister formation. Though they are usually found on the sides of the fingers, ankles, knees, shoulders and over the greater trochanters and iliac crests they may also form on the ears and malar region. Such blisters were formerly thought to be diagnostic of barbiturate poisoning but have now been described in association with such a wide variety of drug intoxications that they should be regarded as non-specific.

Sweating

Salicylate overdosage is the likeliest explanation for excessive sweating after poisoning but infection and hypoglycaemia should be sought and treated if present.

Urinary features

Urinary symptoms after poisoning are seldom encountered. Retention of urine is common after overdosage with anticholinergic drugs, but the patients are usually unconscious or too drowsy to complain of difficulty in micturating. Anuria is usually due to acute tubular necrosis and may be caused by numerous poisons. Polyuria occurs during recovery from tubular necrosis or may be due to lithium-induced diabetes insipidus.

Auditory symptoms

Tinnitus and deafness are common complaints after salicylate poisoning and are present in virtually every adult whose plasma salicylate concentration exceeds 30 mg/dl. These symptoms also occur after quinine poisoning but this is very uncommon.

Temperature disturbances

Hypothermia

Hypothermia (rectal temperature <35°C) commonly occurs after overdosage with CNS depressant drugs, especially alcohol and phenothiazines, and its incidence increases with increasing depth of coma. Environmental temperature is obviously important, but severe hypothermia can occur even in summer.

Fever

Fever may complicate poisoning with substances which:

1. Uncouple oxidative phosphorylation (usually salicylates).
2. Have anticholinergic effects.
3. Cause a generalised increase in neuromuscular activity (sympathomimetic drugs and monoamine oxidase inhibitors).

Fever due to salicylates and anticholinergic drugs is more common in childhood than adult poisoning. Body temperature usually increases spontaneously as consciousness is regained and during recovery it may rise above normal in the absence of infection or tissue necrosis. Fever is not in itself an indication for antibiotics.

EXCLUSION OF OTHER CAUSES OF COMA

General considerations

When the history and circumstantial evidence strongly suggest that coma is due to poisoning there is generally little need for more than a careful physical examination to exclude other causes. Sometimes, however, the diagnosis of poisoning may be considerably less secure and care must be exercised in excluding other pathology. The differential diagnosis of coma is extremely wide and detailed discussion here would be inappropriate. Fortunately many conditions, including meningitis, trauma, hypoglycaemia, diabetic ketoacidosis, uraemia, hepatic encephalopathy and most cerebrovascular accidents, are unlikely to be confused with poisoning by an experienced clinician. On the other hand encephalitis, subarachnoid haemorrhage, brain stem vascular lesions and subdural and extradural haematomas can cause diagnostic difficulties. Suspicion that coma is not the result of poisoning may be aroused by features in the history, physical examination and by the clinical course during the first few hours after admission to hospital.

History

A history of premonitory headache, behaviour changes, nausea and vomiting for a few hours or days before becoming unconscious strongly suggests the presence of an aneurysm, encephalitis or mass lesion within the skull, particularly if there also have been focal neurological symptoms. Any possibility of recent head injury should stimulate a search for evidence of traumatic intracranial haemorrhage.

Examination

Abrasions and lacerations of the scalp increase the possibility of a subdural or extradural haemorrhage, especially if there is bleeding from the ears or nose. Extensive bruising of the limbs and trunk may also be associated with these diagnoses since falls in individuals chronically intoxicated with alcohol or psychotropic drugs can lead to intracranial damage.

Inequality of pupil size is usually considered to be a particularly ominous sign but, found in isolation, is not necessarily an indication of rising intracranial pressure as it may be due to a Holmes–Adie pupil or instillation of drugs into the conjunctival sac.

Lateralising neurological signs are strongly against a diagnosis of poisoning unless they can be explained by some previous illness, e.g. cerebrovascular accident. Unfortunately, brain stem vascular lesions and subarachnoid haemorrhage may be sufficiently severe to make the patient deeply unconscious without lateralising signs and with hyporeflexia and absent plantar responses. In such cases suspicion may be first aroused when the patient fails to progress as expected were poisoning the cause of coma.

Papilloedema is not a feature of poisoning other than with glutethimide or carbon monoxide unless cerebral oedema has developed following prolonged hypoxia or hypotension.

Clinical course

The great majority of patients with drug-induced coma show significant improvement in conscious level within 12 hours of admission to hospital. Some, particularly with phenobarbitone or ethchlorvynol poisoning, require longer (24–48 hours) and a few may become more deeply unconscious before improving. However, such cases are sufficiently uncommon that failure to improve within 12 hours should raise the possibility of some other cause for coma. Rapid deterioration in consciousness with the development of unilateral pupillary dilation or respiratory arrest is much more likely to be due to some intracranial lesion than to poisoning.

Measures to take

Once the clinical suspicion has been raised that coma is not due to drugs various steps should be taken:

1. Interview the patient's relatives and re-appraise the history.

2. Re-examine the patient frequently with particular attention to the neurological system. This includes repeated retinoscopy looking for signs of early papilloedema or subhyaloid haemorrhage. The optic fundi may be difficult to visualise in many cases if the pupils are small or if central cataracts are present, but with skill and perseverance the optic discs can usually be seen. Never use mydriatics to facilitate retinoscopy as this deprives the clinician of the diagnostic value of spontaneous dilatation of one pupil. The scalp should also be re-examined and the soft tissues in the temporal fossae compared since unilateral swelling may be the result of trauma with a possible skull fracture and extradural haematoma.

3. Skull radiography excludes fractures and shows pineal displacement or, rarely, calcification in an arteriovenous malformation.

4. Perform echo encephalography to detect midline displacement.

5. Send urine and plasma to the laboratory to be screened for drugs. The limitations of this approach are discussed on p. 20.

Further investigation depends on the results of this assessment and may involve consultation with neurologists or neurosurgeons.

LABORATORY INVESTIGATIONS

Haematological and biochemical investigations are often performed on the poisoned patient who is seriously ill. The results may suggest possible poisons in cases where there is doubt about the exact nature of the compound involved, but it must be emphasised that abnormal results are not of direct diagnostic significance.

Examination of urine

Changes in the colour of the urine occasionally occur as a result of acute poisoning.

1. Green or blue urine occurs when proprietary preparations containing methylene blue, such as de Witt's pills, are taken.

2. Orange or orange–red urine is found with overdosage of rifampicin or after treatment of iron poisoning with desferrioxamine.

3. Urine which is grey to black in colour strongly suggests poisoning with compounds containing phenols and cresols, e.g. Lysol, and may be confirmed by the characteristic smell of such compounds in the urine.

4. Primidone may crystallise in the urine as it cools. If the urine is then shaken whorls of shimmering, highly refractile crystals can be seen. On microscopy each crystal can be seen to be a needle-shaped hexagon. Their chemical nature is readily confirmed by simple analytical techniques.

Inspection of blood and plasma

Freshly-drawn venous blood that is chocolate-brown in colour suggests methaemoglobinaemia and possible poisoning with oxidising agents such as chlorates, aniline, nitrates or nomifensine.

Pink or brown discolouration of plasma, assuming the blood

sample was taken with care, suggests haemolysis and possible poisoning with chlorates, nomifensine or arsine.

Haematological and biochemical investigations

The value of the results of various emergency laboratory investigations in indicating specific poisons or groups of poisons is shown in Table 2.1.

Screening for poisons

The purpose of an emergency laboratory drug screen is to identify and quantify poisons amenable to specific treatment in patients who are desperately ill and in whom the exact nature of the poison is uncertain. It should not be used merely to confirm the diagnosis suspected from the history or circumstantial evidence unless a positive result will alter management. Laboratory screens for poisons are often tedious and time-consuming and require considerable expertise. They should not be used as an alternative to detailed questioning of the relatives, ambulance team and family doctor to find out which drugs were available or to a thorough search for and interpretation of abnormal physical signs.

No laboratory screen can be expected to detect all possible poisons and the clinical chemist requires as much guidance as the clinician can provide to help direct his analyses. It is, therefore essential that requests for drug screens should be discussed beforehand by the clinician and the laboratory staff. Remember that laboratory staff engaged in prolonged and pointless drug screens cannot at the same time be expected to provide the urgent and much more useful clinical chemistry service often necessary for the management of severely poisoned patients.

When a drug screen is requested the laboratory should be provided with samples of gastric aspirate and urine as well as blood. Drugs and their metabolites are usually present in aspirate and urine in much higher concentrations than in blood, and urine usually has the advantage of being available in larger volumes. Although the urine may be used for identification of the poisons only their concentrations in plasma or blood are useful for management and prognosis.

TABLE 2.1 Diagnostic pointers from emergency laboratory investigations in acute poisoning.

Laboratory finding	Possible toxic causes
Haematology	
Leukocytosis	Of no diagnostic value—common with poisons which cause tissue necrosis
Leukopenia ⎫ Thrombocytopenia ⎬	Colchicine and other cytotoxic drugs
Prothrombin time prolongation	Hepatotoxins (paracetamol, carbon tetrachloride, phenylbutazone, isoniazid, phalloidin) and oral anticoagulants (warfarin and coumarins)
Urea and electrolytes	
Uraemia	Of little differential diagnostic value
Hyperkalaemia	Cardiac glycosides, chloroquine, beta-adrenergic blockers, potassium salts, haemolysis
Hypokalaemia	Diuretics, sympathomimetic drugs
Bicarbonate reduced	Of some diagnostic value, if marked, carry out arterial blood gas analysis
Arterial blood gas analysis	
Metabolic acidosis	Methanol, ethylene glycol, salicylates (rarely), cyanide, phenformin, isoniazid
Respiratory acidosis (or mixed respiratory/ metabolic acidosis)	CNS depressant drugs
Respiratory alkalosis (or mixed respiratory alkalosis/metabolic acidosis)	Salicylates, 2,4D and related compounds, LSD, sympathomimetics
Glucose	
Hypoglycaemia	Insulin, oral hypoglycaemic agents, ethanol, salicylates. May also complicate severe toxic hepatic necrosis
Hyperglycaemia	Drugs causing hepatic necrosis

RADIOLOGY

Radiology is of very limited diagnostic value in acute poisoning. Only a very small proportion of pharmaceutical preparations are radio-opaque, but iron and sustained-release potassium tablets may be visible on an abdominal radiograph. It may also be possible to confirm the ingestion of petroleum distillates on an abdominal film taken in the erect position. The hydrocarbon forms a faintly radio-opaque layer between normal gastric contents and the gas above.

A chest radiograph showing pulmonary oedema in a poisoned patient suggests overdosage with opiates, salicylates or ethchlor-vynol. Similar appearances may be found after inhalation of gases such as chlorine or the oxides of nitrogen, but in these cases the interval between poisoning and development of pulmonary oedema is measured in hours rather than in minutes.

POINTS OF EMPHASIS

- Diagnosis of poisoning is made from the history and circumstantial evidence in the majority of cases.

- Patients' statements about the nature and quantity of drugs ingested must be accepted with caution.

- Poisoning is one of the most common causes of non-traumatic coma in patients under the age of 35 years.

- Isolated symptoms and signs are of no diagnostic value.

- Constellations of symptoms and signs are of diagnostic value.

- Organic brain damage should be suspected if the history of poisoning is unsatisfactory and the depth of coma does not improve within 12 hours.

- Routine biochemical and haematological investigations may rarely suggest a diagnosis of acute poisoning.

- Requests for drug screens should always be discussed with laboratory staff.

- Gastric aspirate and urine are often more useful for drug screens than blood or plasma.

- Abdominal radiographs may occasionally reveal evidence of ingestion of iron and potassium preparations.

CHAPTER 3

General plan for the management of acute poisoning

The severity of physical illness following acute poisoning varies widely. About 80 per cent of children and adults have minimal symptoms and require correspondingly little medical care. On the other hand, at least half of the remainder are very seriously ill and their recovery depends on the highest standards of medical and nursing care. The majority of the latter have taken CNS depressant drugs and management of coma is a vital part of the general approach to the treatment of poisoning. The following steps should be implemented according to the patient's condition:

1. Ensure that the airway, ventilation and blood pressure are adequate.
2. Assess the level of consciousness.
3. Obtain information about the poison if there is uncertainty about its toxicity or appropriate treatment.
4. Consider whether an antidote is available, appropriate or necessary.
5. Consider the need for measures to prevent the absorption of the poison.
6. Consider whether an emergency drug analysis should be requested.
7. Institute a programme of continuing care.
8. Consider whether it is possible or desirable to attempt to increase the elimination of the poison.

MAINTENANCE OF VITAL FUNCTIONS

In any severely poisoned patient the first priority is to ensure that the airway is patent and that alveolar ventilation and circulation are adequate to maintain life while decisions are being made about further treatment. Although these functions are considered separately, it must be emphasised that they are interdependent.

Airway

Upper airway obstruction is one of the most common causes of death in patients dying from poisoning outside hospital. The establishment of a patent airway automatically improves alveolar ventilation and often restores blood pressure.

1. Remove dental plates, making sure that they are carefully set aside and later labelled and stored for return to the patient when consciousness is regained.

2. Pull the tongue forward.

3. Remove saliva or vomitus from the mouth and pharynx. Ideally this is best achieved using a suction catheter, but in an emergency situation a swab wrapped round a finger is highly effective. When suction is being used it is important to avoid inducing gagging and vomiting. Avoid passing catheters through the nose since trauma to the highly vascular nasal epithelium may cause profuse bleeding and add to the difficulties of keeping the airway clear.

4. Insert an endotracheal tube if the patient is deeply unconscious and the cough reflex is depressed or absent. Adult males and females require tubes of 9.0–9.5 mm and 8.0–8.5 mm respectively. The diameter of tube required for children aged 4–12 years is calculated by the formula:

$$\frac{age}{4} + 4.5$$

The size of the tube does not matter when the patient is being mechanically ventilated but is important during spontaneous ventilation when respiratory effort is increased by a tube that is too small.

The inexperienced may find it easier to use the relatively rigid red-rubber Magill tube. This is acceptable for periods of intubation up to about 12 hours. However, if longer periods of intubation are anticipated a soft-seal, sterile plastic tube should be used in the first place or substituted for a Magill tube at a convenient early moment. Plastic tubes are less irritant to the vocal cords and trachea than rubber ones.

5. Ensure that the tube has not been inserted too far since it may enter the right main bronchus, obstruct the left main bronchus and cause atelectasis of the left lung. This can be avoided if care is taken to use a tube which is not too long and by auscultating the lungs immediately after intubation to check that there is air entry into both sides. A chest X-ray should always be taken and will usually show the position of the tip of the tube in relation to the bifurcation of the trachea.

6. Insert a short oropharyngeal airway if the patient is unconscious but unable to accept or tolerate an endotracheal tube. A size 3 airway is suitable for most small or medium-height adults but some may require a size 4.

7. Turn the patient into the semi-prone or three-quarters prone position. If an endotracheal tube has been inserted, keep the neck slightly flexed to avoid distortion of the curve of the tube and undue pressure on the vocal cords and tracheal wall. If an oropharyngeal tube is being used keep the neck flexed and the head extended with the lower jaw pulled forward to increase the anteroposterior diameter of the larynx.

Ventilation

Emergency measures

The most important aspect of improving ventilation is to establish a patent airway as described above. Once this has been done, however, the rate and/or depth of respiration may still be inadequate and immediate steps must be taken to remedy this situation. Do not wait for the results of arterial blood gas analysis. Outside hospital, start mouth-to-mouth respiration; in hospital use an Ambu bag or Water's cannister via a face mask or endotracheal tube. Oxygen should be given.

Assessment of ventilation

In less urgent circumstances the adequacy of ventilation is best assessed by arterial blood gas analysis. This vital investigation is only as valuable as the care taken in obtaining the sample and assessing the results. Attention should be given to the following details:

1. Ensure at the time of sampling that the blood is arterial and not venous. The only certain way to decide this is to observe the blood pulsating into the syringe. Contrary to popular belief, the origin of the blood cannot be determined from its colour or the results of analysis. Unfortunately the more ill the patient, the greater the difficulty in obtaining an arterial sample and the more crucial the investigation.

2. Use the correct concentration of heparin and use as little as possible. A concentration of 1000 iu/ml is satisfactory and the quantity required to fill the needle and hub of the syringe is more than enough. Excessive quantities significantly alter blood gas tensions and raise the hydrogen ion concentration.

3. Obtain a minimum sample volume of 3 ml to help reduce interference from heparin and air bubbles.

4. Advise the biochemist of the body core temperature if the patient is hypothermic or hyperthermic so that appropriate corrections can be applied to the results.

Measurement of respiratory minute volume by some type of spirometer (e.g. a Wright's spirometer) is of limited value in the assessment of the adequacy of ventilation and has been largely superseded by the ready availability of arterial blood gas analysis in most hospitals.

Ventilation and acid-base disturbances in coma

Patients who are unconscious after overdoses of barbiturates or tricyclic antidepressants, but still self-ventilating, seldom show marked carbon dioxide retention though the Pa,co_2 is often near the upper limit of normal. However, the arterial oxygen tension may be unexpectedly low, particularly in grade 4 coma and to a lesser extent in grade 3 coma, probably due to ventilation/perfusion imbalance (see p. 28 for definition of coma grades). The consequence of combined hypoxia and mild carbon dioxide retention is a rise in arterial hydrogen ion concentration (reduction of pH) due to a mixed metabolic and respiratory acidosis. Under no circumstance should attempts be made to correct the metabolic component of the acid–

base disturbance by infusion of alkali before the Pa,co_2 has been brought within the normal range. Hypoxia can usually be corrected by increasing the oxygen content of inspired air.

Improving ventilation

Establishment of a patent airway is of paramount importance in improving ventilation. In the deeply unconscious patient endotracheal intubation reduces the respiratory physiological dead space by about 60–70 ml and correspondingly increases alveolar ventilation.

If ventilation remains inadequate despite these measures, assisted respiration is necessary. The type of ventilator used will depend on what is available locally and is best chosen in conjunction with anaesthetists. Volume cycled respirators are easier to use than pressure cycled types such as the Bird ventilator and are less likely to lead to hyperventilation and reduction of cardiac output.

Hypotension

It is difficult to define hypotension in acute poisoning. By custom the minimum acceptable systolic blood pressure readings are 80 mmHg in young adults and 90 mmHg in patients aged more than 40 years. However, these values are arbitrary and more reliance should be placed on organ perfusion as assessed by the patient's mental state (if conscious), skin temperature or hourly urine output (if catheterised). When hypotension is a problem:

1. Clear the airway, improve ventilation and correct hypoxia as this will abolish hypotension in many ill patients.

2. If hypotension persists, elevate the foot of the bed by about 15–20 cm to increase the venous return to the heart. This simple manoeuvre is effective in the great majority of cases.

In those who fail to respond expand a central venous pressure line and insert the intravascular volume with plasma or dextran.

Rarely, hypotension may remain a serious problem despite these measures and may only improve when some procedure is instituted to remove poison from the circulation (e.g. charcoal haemoperfusion).

ASSESSMENT OF THE LEVEL OF CONSCIOUSNESS

Various methods of grading the level of consciousness of poisoned patients are in use. The Edinburgh method is recommended because it is simple and the grades of coma defined correlate with other features of poisoning including the presence of hypotension, hypothermia and depression of the cough reflex and respiration. Classification is based on the response to commands and pain.

Grade 0   Fully conscious
Grade 1   Drowsy but obeys commands
Grade 2   Unresponsive to commands but responds well to pain
Grade 3   Unresponsive to commands and minimally responsive to pain
Grade 4   Completely unresponsive

Squeezing the rim of the ear is an adequate painful stimulus. Rubbing the sternum with the knuckles is not advised since frequent repetition soon leads to bruising and oedema. By definition, patients in grades 2, 3 and 4 are unconscious. Assessment of level of consciousness should be delayed until the airway and ventilation are satisfactory.

POISONS INFORMATION SERVICES

No doctor could be expected to know the constituents of the infinite array of drugs, household products and agricultural and industrial preparations that may be involved in poisoning episodes, far less their toxic effects and appropriate treatment. Poisons information centres were established to provide such information and to advise on treatment. Any doctor dealing with a poisoned patient is strongly advised to contact the nearest centre if he is in any doubt about the nature or toxicity and the best treatment for the particular poison. The telephone numbers of the United Kingdom centres are given in Appendix 2 (p. 215). If maximum benefit is to be obtained from an enquiry it is important to appreciate the limitations of these services.

1. The organisation and expertise available varies considerably from one information service to another. An enquiry may initially

be answered by a nurse, secretary, pharmacist, information officer or doctor, none of whom necessarily has special knowledge or clinical experience of poisoning. They will consult the appropriate register and read out the constituents and toxic effects of the poison and the recommended treatment. Inevitably, the amount of information given is often limited and general in nature, and if it does not meet the needs, the enquirer should not hesitate to ask to speak to medical staff with practical experience of poisoning.

2. Make certain that you and the person answering the call are in no doubt about the correct spelling of the name of the poison or product. Failure to do so may prevent available information being found or result in misleading and potentially dangerous advice being given.

3. Give the brand name of the drug or commercial product whenever possible. There may be more than one toxic ingredient and you may not necessarily identify the most important one from the list of constituents. Moreover the concentration of the same toxin in different products may vary from insignificant to potentially very dangerous.

4. If you do not know the precise name of the poison but know its purpose (e.g. drain cleaner, dry cleaning agent, bleach, etc.) an enquiry in these general terms may still be worthwhile.

5. Do not be dismayed if information about the poison is sketchy or not available as is frequently the case with uncommon chemicals and industrial compounds. The lack of information simply reflects the rarity of poisoning.

6. Do not expect poisons information services to identify plants and mushrooms from descriptions given over the telephone. These must be identified by the enquirer.

7. Do not ask patients or their relatives to telephone the poisons information centre. It is policy in the United Kingdom to give information only to medically qualified enquirers since telling an already worried patient or parent the features of poisoning might only increase anxiety. It is also arguable that only doctors can assess the seriousness of poisoning and the need for treatment. Much of the information on commercial products is given to the service on a confidential basis and cannot be disclosed to the public.

8. Beware of acting on information obtained through middle parties. The more serious the poisoning episode the more important it is for the doctor involved to personally ask for advice. Do not leave this task to nurses, secretaries or pharmacists who are not trained to

discuss clinical complexities or the relative merits of different forms of treatment.

9. Please answer any request from the information service for details of the course and outcome of a poisoning you have managed. This may be the only way that knowledge of poisoning with new or uncommon compounds can be obtained.

It must be emphasised that poisons information centres exist to provide advice, not to make decisions. Only the doctor managing the patient is in a position to fully assess the clinical situation.

ANTIDOTES

The administration of antidotes to certain poisons can occasionally produce dramatic and life-saving improvement in a patient's condition and obviate the need for protracted intensive care. However, contrary to popular belief, antidotes are available for only a very small number of poisons, most of which are uncommon in everyday clinical practice. They are listed with their appropriate antidotes in Table 3.1 together with the mode of action of the antidotes. Details about use are given under the specific poisons.

PREVENTING ABSORPTION OF POISONS

Emptying the stomach

Emptying the stomach has long been an integral part of the treatment of poisoning with substances which have been ingested. It can be achieved by inducing emesis or by gastric aspiration and lavage. Argument about the relative merits of these methods has detracted from the study of the value of each, in terms of the quantities of drugs recovered. In many cases the apparent amount of drug in the vomitus or lavage fluid hardly seems sufficient to justify the procedure and it has been suggested that gastric emptying is carried out too often. Doubt has also been cast on the efficiency of the methods by reports of large quantities of drug being found in the upper alimentary tract at post-mortem despite apparently successful emptying of the stomach during life. In most of these cases too small a tube has been used or the drug has formed a large concretion.

TABLE 3.1   Antidotes.

Poisons	Antidote	Mode of action
Anticholinergic compounds	Physostigmine salicylate	Cholinesterase inhibitor
Anticoagulants (oral)	Vitamin K_1	Pharmacological antagonist
	Fresh frozen plasma Clotting factors	Replacement of missing clotting factors
β-adrenergic blockers	Isoprenaline	Pharmacological antagonist
	Glucagon	Stimulates myocardial adenocyclase
Cyanide	Dicobalt edetate	Chelating agents
Ethylene glycol	Ethanol	Competitive substrate for alcohol dehydrogenase
Heavy metals	Dimercaprol Penicillamine	Chelating agents
Iron salts	Desferrioxamine	Chelating agent
Methanol	Ethanol	Competitive substrate for alcohol dehydrogenase
Narcotic analgesics	Naloxone	Pharmacological antagonist
Organophosphate insecticides	Atropine	Acetylcholine antagonist
	Pralidoxime	Cholinesterase reactivator
Paracetamol	N-acetylcysteine Methionine Cysteamine	? SH donors or glutathione precursors
Pentazocine	Naloxone	Pharmacological antagonist
Sympathomimetics	β-adrenergic blockers	Pharmacological antagonist
Thallium	Prussian blue	Chelating agent

However, in others there is no doubt that large amounts of drug are recovered and that emptying the stomach makes a valuable contribution to reducing the severity and duration of poisoning. Unfortunately the value of lavage can only be assessed after it has been done.

When to empty the stomach

The dilemma of identifying the patients most likely to benefit from gastric emptying is unlikely ever to be resolved and hard and fast rules cannot be laid down. Instead, make a decision after considering the following:

1. *Has a dangerous compound been ingested?* It is obvious that the more toxic the poison, the more important it is to retrieve any

remaining in the stomach. In contrast, relatively innocuous compounds (e.g. oral contraceptive preparations, benzodiazepines) make it less necessary to empty the stomach.

2. *Has a dangerous quantity been ingested?* Some poisons (e.g. cyanide and some formulations of paraquat) are potentially lethal in even very small quantities and make it mandatory to empty the stomach. Others have to be taken in large amounts before they are likely to be dangerous. Danger has to be assessed, not only in terms of life or death, but also in terms of the severity and duration of toxic effects. The amount likely to be dangerous will clearly vary according to the weight of the patient. Assessment of the risk may require considerable experience.

Doctors are frequently anxious to know the 'fatal dose' of a poison but the outcome of poisoning may depend on complications which are unpredictable (e.g. inhalation of vomit) or only occur in a small proportion of patients (e.g. convulsions, cardiac dysrhythmias). As has already been pointed out, it is frequently impossible to be certain how much has been taken. Knowing the 'fatal dose' may be a comfort to the doctor but may induce a false sense of security and result in failure to empty the stomach when it might be advantageous to do so. Conversely others may err on the safe side and overuse gastric emptying. Fortunately a decision about emptying the stomach seldom has to be made on the quantity ingested alone. In doubtful cases advice can be obtained from the poisons information services.

3. *How long since ingestion?* The time since ingestion is important in determining how much drug is likely to be in the stomach and available for recovery. The rate at which the stomach empties is increased by previous gastric surgery and delayed when the patient is unconscious. However in most circumstances there is unlikely to be benefit in emptying the stomach if longer than 4 hours has elapsed since ingestion.

4. *Has the poison altered the rate of gastric emptying?* The poison itself can reduce or accelerate the rate of gastric emptying. Drugs such as metoclopramide and irritant poisons such as paraquat probably increase the rate of gastric emptying while anticholinergic compounds and narcotics delay emptying and increase the time during which gastric emptying may be beneficial. Even with the latter, however, there is probably nothing to be gained from emptying the stomach after 6 hours have elapsed since ingestion. It has been suggested that salicylates cause pyloric spasm and that significant quantities may be retrieved up to 24 hours from ingestion

but the evidence is unconvincing and the same guide-lines probably apply to salicylates as to other drugs.

5. *Is the patient unconscious?* As coma becomes deeper bowel sounds tend to disappear and it is assumed that gastric emptying is delayed as part of the overall reduction in gut activity. It is therefore recommended that gastric aspiration and lavage be carried out in every unconscious poisoned patient if the airway can be protected.

6. *Can the airway be protected?* Emptying the stomach, whether by inducing emesis or by lavage tube, is only safe if the respiratory passages can be protected. The patient therefore must have an adequate cough reflex or be sufficiently depressed that a cuffed endotracheal tube can be inserted. To persist with gastric lavage in a patient who cannot cough adequately yet is too 'light' to accept an endotracheal tube is to invite acute respiratory obstruction or aspiration pneumonia. In such cases review the clinical situation at half-hourly intervals; if the level of consciousness deteriorates it may become possible to intubate and carry out lavage with safety and if it improves gastric emptying is clearly unnecessary.

7. *Has a petroleum distillate been taken?* Petroleum distillates (long-chain hydrocarbons) can cause serious pneumonia if aspirated into the lungs. Unless large enough amounts have been ingested it is customary to recommend that gastric emptying, by any method, should be avoided (p. 172).

Emesis or lavage?

The stomach can be emptied either by inducing vomiting or by passing a gastric lavage tube. It is doubtful if one is any more efficient than the other in recovering drugs and neither can be relied upon to empty the stomach completely. The method adopted will depend on the age, conscious level and degree of co-operation of the patient and the facilities and expertise available.

Gastric aspiration and lavage is indicated for all unconscious patients and most adults who will co-operate. Induced emesis is the method of choice for children since a large enough tube cannot be passed and emesis is generally accepted as being psychologically less traumatic than passing a gastric tube. It should also be used in adults in whom gastric emptying is indicated but who refuse gastric lavage.

Induced emesis

The most satisfactory method of inducing emesis is to give 15–30 ml of syrup of ipecacuanha followed by 200 ml of water. This will make about 70 per cent of patients vomit within 20 minutes. If ineffective, the dose can be repeated after this time with success in a further 20 per cent.

The use of salt and water to induce vomiting is unreliable and largely ineffective but still widely practised by doctors and members of the public when confronted by someone who has ingested a poison. In most cases the emetic does no harm but in others, anxious relatives, eager to ensure rapid retrieval of the poison, may give grossly excessive quantities of salt and cause severe hypernatraemia. Several adults and children have died as a result and in many other deaths the role of salt may not have been appreciated. The use of saline emetics is therefore deprecated. Mechanical methods are inefficient and tartar emetic and copper sulphate solutions are potentially lethal.

Gastric aspiration and lavage

The best results are obtained from gastric aspiration and lavage by the following technique:

1. Before starting ensure that powerful suction apparatus is present and functioning. This may be required to remove gastric contents regurgitated around the stomach tube and should be capable of coping with large volumes in quite short periods of time.
2. Lie the patient in the left lateral position on a trolley.
3. Raise the foot of the trolley by 15–20 cm.
4. Lubricate and pass a Jacques stomach tube (size 30 English gauge, external diameter approximately 14 mm) into the stomach. This size of tube is sufficiently large to be unlikely to pass through the vocal cords and is sufficiently firm (without being inflexible) to be passed without much co-operation from the patient. Confirm its position in the stomach by aspirating or blowing some air down the tube while auscultating over the stomach. Use disposable plastic stomach tubes for drug addicts or others suspected of having had hepatitis.
5. Siphon off the gastric contents before carrying out lavage.
6. Perform gastric lavage by connecting the tube to a large funnel

(using 1 metre rubber or plastic hose) and by pouring 300 ml aliquots of tepid tap water down the stomach tube and then siphoning it off. Repeat the procedure until the returning fluid is clear of tablet particles. The efficiency of this technique may be improved by gently massaging over the left hypochondrium to aid the dislodgement and mixing of tablet fragments trapped in mucosal folds.

7. Once the effluent is clear withdraw the tube, taking care to occlude it completely between the fingers so that fluid left in the tube will not flood out when the end leaves the oesophagus and enters the pharynx. This simple measure should help reduce the danger of aspiration into the lungs. The suction apparatus may be needed.

Complications

Oesophageal rupture. Rupture of the oesophagus is a potentially fatal complication of gastric lavage but is extremely uncommon. It may be avoided by attention to the following:

1. Never carry out gastric lavage without good reason.
2. Use a lavage tube which has a rounded end and which is made of a soft, flexible material and yet is sufficiently firm to be passed without too much co-operation from the patient. Rubber tubes (size 30 English gauge) are ideal. Particular care must be taken when using plastic tubes which tend to be less flexible and when 'breaking-in' new rubber tubes.
3. Lubricate the tube well with KY jelly.
4. Do not use force to pass the tube. Oesophageal perforation is most likely to occur when the patient is struggling. If the patient is unco-operative to this extent the need for gastric lavage should be reconsidered or sedation given before trying again.

Following oesophageal perforation the patient may complain of central chest pain and rapidly becomes shocked with sweating, pallor, tachycardia and hypotension. Crepitus may be palpable in the root of the neck and subcutaneous and mediastinal emphysema may be seen on the chest X-ray. Fluids by mouth should be forbidden while an urgent contrast X-ray of the oesophagus is arranged to identify the point of rupture. Oesophagoscopy and closure of the perforation will be required and the advice and help of a thoracic surgeon should be sought immediately.

Inhalation of gastric contents. Inhalation of gastric contents is an ever-present hazard in unconscious patients. The risk may be reduced by observing the following:

1. Keep the patient in the semi-prone or three-quarters prone position with the head slightly dependent during transport to hospital and under no circumstances allow an unconscious patient to lie on his back.

2. Never give ipecac to patients likely to lose consciousness rapidly.

3. If the cough reflex is impaired, insert a cuffed endotracheal tube before attempting gastric lavage.

4. Always ensure that powerful suction apparatus, capable of removing large volumes of regurgitated fluid and particulate material, is available and functioning before starting gastric lavage.

5. Take care to occlude the lumen of a lavage tube before withdrawing it because fluid remaining in the lumen may flood into the pharynx and be inhaled as the end of the tube emerges from the oesophagus.

The pulmonary response to inhalation of gastric content depends on several factors, including the volume inhaled, the pH of the fluid and the presence and size of food particles.

Experimental evidence indicates that the morbidity and mortality is particularly high when the pH of the aspirated fluid is less than 2.5. Acid fluid damages the lungs instantly and they rapidly become oedematous and haemorrhagic with areas of atelectasis due to reduced surfactant activity. Respiratory effort increases, bronchospasm may develop and arterial blood gas analysis usually shows a mixed respiratory and metabolic acidosis with hypoxaemia.

Inhalation of large food particles occasionally causes rapid death from laryngeal or tracheal obstruction whereas smaller particles cause lobar or segmental collapse. The role played by non-obstructing food particles in producing pulmonary damage is poorly understood but animal studies clearly demonstrate their ability to produce an extensive haemorrhagic pneumonia even when pH is neutral.

Treatment of laryngeal or major bronchus obstruction is a matter of the utmost urgency and laryngoscopy or bronchoscopy may be required to remove large food particles. However, bronchoscopy is hazardous in acutely hypoxic patients and is best avoided unless there is clear evidence of obstruction of a major airway. There is no evidence that bronchial lavage is helpful. In less severe cases it is usually sufficient to insert an endotracheal tube and carry out frequent bronchial suction which has the advantage of inducing coughing and thereby facilitates clearance of food fragments. It will not reduce the immediate pulmonary damage caused by acid and non-obstructing food particles. Frequent physiotherapy is essential.

Hypoxia may be corrected by increasing the inspired oxygen concentration but when severe, or associated with hypercapnia, assisted ventilation with or without positive end-expiratory pressure may be required. The most suitable method for individual cases is best decided in conjunction with anaesthetists.

It is traditional to give corticosteroids to patients who have inhaled gastric contents in the hope that pulmonary damage will be reduced but there is no convincing evidence that they are beneficial.

Other supportive measures, including bronchodilators for bronchospasm and intravenous fluids for hypovolaemia, may be required. Antibiotics should be withheld until there is clear evidence of infection and an organism has been isolated.

Lipid pneumonia. The ingestion of petroleum distillate (long-chain hydrocarbon) contained in paraffin, petrol, kerosene, turpentine substitute and furniture polishes may be complicated by aspiration into the lungs. The resulting acute inflammatory reaction in the alveoli and interstitial tissues is commonly referred to as a lipid or lipoid pneumonia. The hydrocarbon is phagocytosed by macrophages and can be identified in their cytoplasmic vacuoles.

The severity of symptoms caused by lipoid pneumonia is variable and there is no specific treatment. Antibiotics and corticosteroids have been recommended but the evidence for their efficacy is unconvincing. Whether the incidence of lipoid pneumonia can be minimised by not attempting to empty the stomach is controversial (p. 172).

Activated charcoal

In some countries activated charcoal is widely used for the first-aid treatment of acute poisoning. It is manufactured from a variety of materials which are heated in the absence of air until carbon is formed. The carbon is then 'activated', usually by exposing it to steam at high temperatures. This produces pores and channels throughout the particles and greatly increases the surface area available for adsorption of drugs and chemicals.

Administration of activated charcoal within minutes of ingestion considerably reduces the absorption of drugs, occasionally this may be by as much as 90 per cent. However, if administration is delayed for an hour or more, the ability of activated charcoal to prevent absorption is greatly reduced. Its efficacy is also decreased by the presence of food in the stomach.

The role of activated charcoal in the treatment of poisoning is also limited by its acceptability to patients. About ten times as much charcoal must be given as there is drug to be adsorbed and doses of 50–100 g are necessary.

Activated charcoal may be of value in the management of accidental poisoning in children but adults usually present too long after overdosage for it to be useful. It may, however, be given regularly over a period of a few days to interrupt the entero-hepatic circulation of some drugs which have long plasma half-lives (e.g. phenobarbitone and cardiac glycosides).

Syrup of ipecac should not be given after activated charcoal since the emetine will be adsorbed and be ineffective.

'Universal' antidote (activated charcoal, magnesium oxide and tannic acid) should never be used.

Whole gut lavage

Whole gut lavage is a method of evacuating the bowel contents rapidly. It involves passing a naso-gastric tube and instilling warm, normal saline into the stomach at a rate of 2 l/h. Watery diarrhoea soon develops and within 2–3 hours faecal material is usually absent from the rectal effluent. This procedure has been recommended for the treatment of poisoning with paraquat and slow release drug formulations, particularly when the latter have passed into the small bowel and are beyond recovery by gastric emptying. The value of this treatment has not been adequately assessed. Patients usually tolerate it well but hypokalaemia may develop.

EMERGENCY DRUG ANALYSIS

A venous blood sample should be taken for toxicological analysis from every patient admitted because of poisoning, the only exceptions being drug addicts or patients who may be Australia antigen positive. In the latter case blood should only be taken if mandatory for the management of the poisoning and provided that appropriate precautions are taken to protect the person carrying out the procedure and the laboratory staff. If venesection is necessary in such patients a sample should be taken simultaneously for screening for Australia antigen.

There are two main reasons for taking blood for drug analysis:

1. In the important minority, to assess the severity of poisoning and to indicate the need for specific treatment.

2. For legal purposes should the patient die or develop some unexpected complication. It is therefore vital that the samples are accurately labelled with the patient's name, the date and time (24-hour clock) and kept refrigerated till the patient is discharged.

It will usually suffice to take 10 ml of blood into a lithium heparin tube. There are two exceptions to this rule: a plain tube must be used if it is intended to measure lithium concentrations, and blood for carboxyhaemoglobin estimations is best taken into heparinised syringes taking care to exclude air. With lithium heparin samples it is preferable, if possible, to separate the plasma and store it at $-20\,°C$ if analysis is to be delayed.

In the vast majority of poisonings there is no justification for requesting an emergency drug analysis. It is common clinical practice to measure plasma concentrations of barbiturates routinely in unconscious patients but these investigations are done more to confirm the diagnosis and comfort the doctor than to alter management of the patient. Knowledge of the plasma barbiturate concentration is highly unlikely to make the clinician do anything more than continue to support vital functions. Salicylates rarely cause coma in adults and in the absence of other clinical features of salicylism, particularly hyperventilation, significant salicylate poisoning is unlikely. Requests for emergency drug analyses should be restricted to those poisonings where specific treatment is available and the need for it is determined from the plasma drug concentration. These include paracetamol, salicylate, iron, lithium and paraquat. Measurement of plasma drug concentrations is mandatory before attempting to enhance elimination by forced diuresis, haemodialysis or haemoperfusion. All unconscious poisoned patients should be screened for paracetamol since patients have recovered from sedative overdoses only to become jaundiced and die from hepatic failure. Such deaths might have been avoided had the early analysis of blood led to administration of specific treatment. Screening unconscious adults for paracetamol ingestion is far more important than looking for salicylates but, paradoxically, is much less commonly requested.

CONTINUING CARE

Once emergency measures have been taken to maintain vital functions, the stomach has been emptied and antidotes, if available, have been administered, unconscious patients will require continuing intensive care. Their survival depends more on the standard of nursing care than on medical technology.

Respiratory care

General

Every unconscious patient should be nursed in the semi-prone or three-quarters prone position. It is vital that the back frame of the bed should be removed at the outset, or be capable of being removed without difficulty, to allow immediate access for endotracheal intubation.

Secretions which collect in the oropharynx and especially in the dependent cheek should be removed regularly by suction. It is particularly important to do this before turning the patient from one side to the other to prevent aspiration of buccal secretions into the trachea. Removal of secretions in the mouth and pharynx is usually done blindly but if a rattle persists in the upper airway, direct laryngosopy should be carried out to remove remaining secretions under direct vision.

Oropharyngeal tubes should be removed and inspected at 4-hour intervals and replaced if there is evidence that they are becoming blocked with secretions.

Intubated patients

If the patient has an endotracheal tube *in situ*, regular bronchial suction should be carried out using a sterile technique according to the amount of secretions to be removed. It is absolutely vital that the inspired air is adequately humidified and warmed to avoid drying and crusting of the tracheal mucosa and of secretions lying in the tube. The type of humidifier to be used should be decided in consultation with the anaesthetists. The importance of using plastic endotracheal tubes if intubation is required for longer than 12 hours has already been emphasised (p. 25). The endotracheal tube should be removed once the patient starts to gag or have paroxysms of coughing and should be replaced by an oropharyngeal airway.

Daily samples of bronchial aspirate should be sent for bacteriological examination for as long as the patient is intubated. Antibiotics should not be given prophylactically to unconscious patients. A daily chest radiograph should be taken while the patient is unconscious or as indicated by the development of some respiratory complication.

Complications

Obstruction of endotracheal tubes. Endotracheal tubes may become obstructed in several ways including mechanical distortion, herniation of the inflated cuff over the end and by inspissation of secretions in the lumen. The last named can be prevented by carrying out regular bronchial suction and humidifying the inspired air while herniation of the cuff is highly unlikely if it is not over-inflated. Kinking of the tube may be minimised by keeping the patient's neck slightly flexed.

Obstruction of the tube will cause a marked increase in inspiratory effort with indrawing of the intercostal spaces, soft tissues in the root of the neck and, in younger patients, the lower sternum. Central cyanosis will be present. Deflate the cuff and withdraw the tube immediately.

Aspiration pneumonia. Unconscious patients often aspirate pharyngeal secretions and are unable to clear them because the cough reflex is depressed. They are therefore likely to develop an aspiration pneumonia. This complication is usually suspected from the findings on clinical examination of the lungs, fever or purulent bronchial secretions and is confirmed by chest radiography. A Gram film of bronchial aspirate should be made and appropriate antibiotic therapy begun before the results of culture are available. If no organism is obvious on the direct film a broad spectrum antibiotic such as ampicillin should be given and changed later if necessary.

Frequent bronchial suction and intensive physiotherapy are mandatory. Bronchoscopy should be reserved for patients with lobar collapse.

If respiratory infection is severe and life-threatening, consider methods of shortening the duration of coma in order to speed the return of an effective cough reflex.

Skin care

Unconscious patients should be turned from one side to the other at 2-hour intervals or more frequently if skin lesions are present. Careful attention must be given to skin over bony prominences to avoid pressure sores.

Bullous lesions should be kept intact for as long as possible to reduce the likelihood of infection, but once they burst, the roof should be removed and the denuded area covered with a sterile, absorbent, non-stick dressing until exudation stops. The dressing should be replaced daily or more frequently, depending on the amount of discharge. When the discharge stops or is minimal the area should be left exposed to dry and crust over.

Eye care

Blinking is abolished in unconscious patients and great care must be taken to ensure that the eyelids are kept closed, taping them down if necessary, to avoid exposure keratitis. Instillation of methylcellulose eye drops into the conjunctival sac, three or four times daily, will also be helpful.

Some patients who are kept lying horizontally without pillows, or who have been nursed in a head-down position because of hypotension, rapidly develop marked subconjunctival, eyelid and facial oedema. This may be the result of posture but a drug effect on blood vessels may also contribute. It is of little importance in itself but may reflect a tendency to oedema in the upper respiratory tract and, if the blood pressure permits, the head should be raised above body level, preferably by tilting the whole bed.

Fluid balance

Many patients (e.g. those poisoned with benzodiazepines and tricyclic antidepressants) do not require intravenous fluids since most are able to take oral fluids within 12–24 hours. However, in severely poisoned patients a venous line should be inserted in case urgent drug therapy is necessary. The temptation to give large volumes of intravenous fluids must be resisted. Barbiturates, narcotics and other CNS depressants have antidiuretic effects and unconscious, hypoventilating and hypothermic patients have reduced insensible fluid losses. It is therefore unnecessary to give more than 2 litres of fluid intravenously in 24 hours unless an attempt is being made to force a diuresis. Nor is there any need to start until the patient has been unconscious for 24 hours. When maintenance fluids are indicated 5% dextrose (1.0 litre) and 0.9% saline (0.5 litre) in rotation are usually adequate but should be altered as indicated by the plasma electrolytes.

Bladder care

The bladder in most unconscious patients can usually be emptied by applying firm suprapubic pressure. The great majority of poisoned adults admitted in coma will be conscious within 12 hours, will produce relatively little urine during that time and will not be grateful to find themselves catheterised unnecessarily. Catheterisation is indicated when:

1. There is considerable bladder distension which cannot be emptied by fundal pressure.
2. Renal failure is suspected.
3. A forced diuresis is being undertaken.

Hypothermia

Simple measures

Hypothermia is seldom severe and the rectal temperature rarely falls below 30 °C. Usually only simple measures are required for its correction and there is no virtue in attempting rapid correction in acute poisoning. The patient should be nursed in a normally warm room and covered with a reasonable number of blankets. It is customary to wrap the patient in a sheet of aluminiumised plastic to reflect back radiant heat from the body but this type of covering is no more efficient than ordinary plastic sheeting. The latter is therefore useful in the first-aid situation. The efficiency of both materials is reduced if moisture condenses on the inner aspect of the sheet and this can be minimised by placing a blanket between the patient and the plastic cover. It is important that hypothermic patients are unwrapped for as short periods as possible and to the least extent for nursing and medical procedures. These measures, together with warming the inspired air through a humidifier, will usually produce a slow return of body temperature to normal.

Other measures

Various more elaborate techniques have been used to correct hypothermia. These include heating one forearm in a water bath at 37 °C or using a soda lime cannister as a heat exchanger to warm inspired air. In extreme cases haemodialysis or irrigation of the mediastinum or peritoneal cavity with warm fluids have been used but it is very doubtful if such heroic measures can ever be justified for the treatment of hypothermia alone. Body temperature usually rises as the level of consciousness improves and patients whose hypothermia is refractory to simple treatment are likely to be severely poisoned or elderly. Procedures to enhance elimination of the poison may be indicated.

INCREASING ELIMINATION OF POISONS

General considerations

Various techniques have been used in attempts to enhance the elimination of poisons, including exchange transfusion, forced diuresis, peritoneal dialysis, haemodialysis and, more recently, haemoperfusion through charcoal and ion exchange resins, and plasmapheresis. Unfortunately, the enthusiasm with which they have been advocated has not always been founded on critical appraisal of their efficacy. All too frequently the claims for their value are based on the recovery of the patient after treatment without any attempt to identify the drug, far less quantify the amount removed or its clearance by the procedure. Even when such attempts have been made the analytical methods have frequently been non-specific, measuring inactive metabolites as well as active drug, with the consequence that the conclusions were misleading.

There is no doubt that techniques to eliminate poisons, particularly forced diuresis, have been used excessively and inappropriately, occasionally with fatal consequences. Clearly they are not indicated in poisoning with compounds for which there is a specific antidote or with those such as benzodiazepines which are relatively harmless in overdosage.

Exchange transfusion is an inefficient method of eliminating poisons and even in childhood has very little place as a therapeutic manoeuvre. Peritoneal dialysis has only about 20 per cent the efficiency of haemodialysis and the amount of drug removed seldom justifies the potential complications of the procedure. The role of plasmapheresis has yet to be defined. When active elimination of a poison is indicated the choice usually lies between forced diuresis, haemodialysis and some form of haemoperfusion.

Forced diuresis

Forced diuresis is the simplest method of enhancing the excretion of some poisons. It increases the renal clearance of compounds which are partly reabsorbed in the renal tubules. Its value can be significantly increased by altering urine pH according to whether the drug is acidic or basic. Alkalinisation of the urine increases ionisation, and thereby prevents reabsorption of acidic compounds such as salicylates, phenobarbitone and phenoxyacetate herbicides. Conversely, acidification of the urine promotes the excretion of basic drugs such as quinine, amphetamines, fenfluramine and phencyclidine.

Forced alkaline diuresis

In clinical practice forced alkaline diuresis is the type commonly required, the usual indications being moderate or severe salicylate and phenobarbitone poisoning. The object is to induce a brisk diuresis by infusing large volumes of fluid intravenously and to alkalinise the urine by including isotonic sodium bicarbonate solution (1.26%) in the infusion regime. The precise rate and duration of the infusion and the amount of alkali given do not matter provided the objectives are achieved without undue risk to the patient. Regimes suitable for salicylate and phenobarbitone poisoning are discussed under these headings.

Patients treated by forced diuresis must have healthy hearts and kidneys if pulmonary oedema, the major complication, is to be avoided. Careful and frequent assessment of fluid balance is mandatory during the procedure and bladder catheterisation is necessary in unconscious patients. However, patients who are conscious do not normally require to be catheterised. If the onset of the diuresis is delayed or if the fluid input exceeds output by more than 2 litres at any time an intravenous diuretic should be given. Urine pH should be measured at frequent intervals using narrow-range indicator paper and the amount of intravenous alkali adjusted to keep pH between 7 and 8. If large amounts of bicarbonate are necessary there is a danger of producing a severe systemic metabolic alkalosis and arterial blood gas analysis should be carried out. Hypokalaemia and hypocalcaemia are well-recognised complications and large quantities of intravenous potassium may be required to keep plasma concentrations within normal limits. Hypocalcaemia usually only reaches serious levels if forced alkaline diuresis is prolonged (>12 h) and 10 ml of 10% calcium gluconate should be given slowly intravenously every 6 hours.

Forced acid diuresis

Forced acid diuresis enhances the elimination of amphetamines, quinine, fenfluramine and phencyclidine but is seldom necessary since severe poisoning with these drugs is uncommon. The diuresis is induced by giving 5% dextrose (1.0 litre) and 0.9% saline (0.5 litre) intravenously in rotation at a rate of 0.5 l/h. Acidification of the urine is achieved by giving ammonium chloride orally or intravenously according to the patient's level of consciousness. The first dose (1.5 g) should be given over 1 hour in the first unit of dextrose. Urine pH should be measured hourly or more frequently using narrow-range indicator paper. Further ammonium chloride is given as necessary to keep urine pH below 5.0.

Fluid balance must be carefully monitored and a diuretic given if output falls behind input by 2 litres or more. Arterial [H^+] and gas tensions should be measured 2-hourly.

Haemodialysis

Haemodialysis is an effective method of increasing the elimination of small molecules (molecular weight <350 daltons) which cross semipermeable membranes readily. Maximum removal of poison depends on the following factors.

1. The plasma concentration of the poison should be high to produce a steep diffusion gradient between plasma and dialyser bath fluid. The common poisons most likely to satisfy this criterion are salicylates, phenobarbitone, ethanol and methanol.

2. Protein and tissue binding of the poison should be as small as possible because the diffusion gradient depends on the plasma concentration of free drug rather than on the total drug concentration.

3. The poison should be water-soluble rather than lipid-soluble. This criterion to some extent explains the success of haemodialysis in removing salicylates and phenobarbitone and its doubtful value in poisoning with barbiturate hypnotics and glutethimide.

4. The volume of distribution of the poison should be as small as possible. Compounds such as lithium and potassium are readily dialysable and plasma concentrations can be reduced rapidly by haemodialysis. Unfortunately their volume of distribution is large so that plasma concentrations quickly rise within a few hours of stopping dialysis. It is therefore preferable to use an alternative treatment.

Most of the serious poisonings encountered in clinical practice are unsuitable for treatment by haemodialysis. Barbiturate hypnotics, glutethimide and methaqualone are poorly dialysable because of their lipid-solubility and tricyclic antidepressants have a large volume of distribution with plasma concentrations too low for haemodialysis to be of value. Haemodialysis still has a role in severe salicylate poisoning and possibly in phenobarbitone poisoning though haemoperfusion is more efficient in the latter.

Haemoperfusion

The ability of activated charcoal to adsorb drugs has been known for many years. It is given orally to reduce the absorption of ingested poisons and was used in the filters of gas masks in the last World War to adsorb various gases. In 1962 a Greek physician published an account of the use of activated charcoal to remove drugs from the blood of poisoned adults.

Technical considerations

The technique is simple. Arterial blood is led from the radial artery to the bottom of a cylinder packed with granules of activated charcoal and primed with saline. The blood is allowed to percolate through the charcoal and is filtered at the top of the cylinder and returned to the patient through a convenient vein. This technique has now been shown to remove a wide variety of drugs, particularly the barbiturate hypnotics and glutethimide which are poorly dialysable, and has the advantages of being more efficient and simpler to use than haemodialysis. Initially, however, it was not without some disadvantages. Hypotension, charcoal embolisation, leukopenia and, more serious, thrombocytopenia were common. Fragmentation and embolisation of charcoal particles has now been eliminated by coating the granules with an acrylic hydrogel at the expense of only a slight reduction in adsorbing capacity. The platelet count falls by 25–50 per cent in the first 2 hours of haemoperfusion but then rises despite continuation of the procedure. Haemorrhagic complications occasionally arise but are uncommon.

More recently ion-exchange resins have been used in place of activated charcoal and clinical experience with two, Amberlite XAD-2 and Amberlite XAD-4, has been published. Amberlite XAD-2 is an uncharged, macroreticular, copolymer which can be autoclaved or gas sterilised and does not fragment easily. Amberlite XAD-4 is chemically identical to XAD-2 but offers twice or more the surface area. Both have a particular affinity for lipid-soluble drugs but, as with activated charcoal, they also adsorb platelets.

Clinical use

There is no doubt that the advent of charcoal and resin haemoperfusion constitutes a major advance in the treatment of severe poisoning with CNS depressant drugs including barbiturate hypnotics, phenobarbitone, glutethimide, methaqualone, ethchlorvynol and meprobamate. Unfortunately, the evidence suggests that these techniques do not remove significant quantities of tricyclic antidepressants. It must be emphasised that haemoperfusion will only be required by a small minority of very severely poisoned patients and it should be regarded as an adjunct to, rather than a substitute for, meticulous supportive care. Patients suitable for charcoal or resin haemoperfusion should satisfy the first and at least one other of the following criteria:

1. The plasma concentration of the drug should not be less than:

phenobarbitone	150 mg/l
barbiturate hypnotics	50
glutethimide	50
methaqualone	40
meprobamate	100
ethchlorvynol	150

2. Poisoning must be clinically severe, with grade 4 coma, hypothermia, hypotension and respiratory depression.

3. The patient's clinical state should be deteriorating or failing to improve despite supportive care.

4. Serious complications should be present, e.g. hepatic and renal insufficiency or extensive pneumonia while the patient is still unconscious.

COMPLICATIONS OF POISONING

Complications occurring during the course of acute poisoning may be due to predictable, but uncommon, effects of the poison or to chance events resulting from impaired consciousness.

Pulmonary oedema

Pulmonary oedema complicating poisoning may be cardiac or non-cardiac in aetiology. The former is far more common and is usually the result of gross fluid overload during forced diuresis. In many cases there is no pharmacokinetic justification for attempting forced diuresis; in others no allowance is made for the possible nephrotoxic or myocardial depressant effects of the poison itself. The antidiuretic effect of some drugs (e.g. narcotics, barbiturates, salicylates and paracetamol) may also be an important aetiological factor. Fatalities occur and are all the more tragic since most are avoidable. This variety of pulmonary oedema should be treated conventionally by stopping fluid administration and giving diuretics and oxygen. If renal failure is present, dialysis may be necessary to remove the excess fluid.

Non-cardiac pulmonary oedema occurs with some inhaled toxins (ammonia, chlorine, oxides of nitrogen) and with ingestion of salicylates, narcotics, paraquat, ethchlorvynol. This form of pulmonary oedema does not respond to diuretics and digoxin but may to corticosteroids which should be given in full doses (hydrocortisone 100 mg 6-hourly by injection or prednisolone 60–80 mg daily orally).

Renal failure

Acute renal failure due to renal tubular necrosis is a relatively uncommon complication of acute poisoning and is usually the result of a combination of hypotension, hypoxia and a predictable direct effect of the poison on tubular cells (e.g. paraquat, salicylate, paracetamol, carbon tetrachloride). The ill-advised use of vasopressor drugs may also contribute and rarely gross intravascular haemolysis or myoglobinuria may be the cause. Even in the absence of these factors, some drugs (e.g. heroin) cause marked, unexplained reduction in effective renal plasma flow and glomerular filtration rate.

Renal failure may be anticipated from the patient's history and condition and strongly suspected when oliguria develops. Urinary retention should always be excluded as a possible cause of apparent oliguria. Urine production should be recorded carefully and 24 hour collections kept for measurement of osmolality and electrolytes. Conscious patients are usually able to void naturally if a large enough volume is present in the bladder. Indiscriminate catheterisation of all unconscious patients cannot be justified, and catheterisation should be reserved for:

1. Patients with retention that cannot be relieved by suprapubic pressure.
2. Those in coma who are undergoing forced diuresis.
3. When there is a strong suspicion of renal failure.

The plasma urea and electrolytes should be measured daily. If there is a likelihood of concurrent hepatocellular damage the plasma creatinine should also be measured since it is a more reliable indicator of renal failure than the urea under these circumstances. The central venous pressure should be assessed by insertion of a central venous line and the intravascular volume expanded with plasma as necessary. It may then be possible to initiate a diuresis by giving frusemide (0.25 or 0.5 g) intravenously over 20 min. Careful fluid balance throughout is mandatory and intake should be adjusted to the urine volume in the preceding 24 hours with an additional 0.5 litre to make up for insensible loss. Most acutely poisoned patients with renal failure are too ill to want to eat and dietary protein restriction is irrelevant. If, despite these measures, the plasma urea or creatinine continues to rise, the patient's blood should be screened for hepatitis-B surface antigen and the patient referred for haemodialysis.

Cerebral oedema

Generalised cerebral oedema is frequently found in fatal cases of acute poisoning and may well be present in others who are desperately ill but survive. It is produced by various factors operating simultaneously including hypoxia and hypercapnia due to respiratory failure, hypotension (the effects of which may have been potentiated by posture), hypoglycaemia and possibly a drug-induced impairment of capillary integrity. The majority of patients who develop cerebral oedema probably do so before admission to hospital though in others it may be the consequence of refractory hypotension or protracted attempts at cardio-respiratory resuscitation. Diagnosis is usually a matter of conjecture but computerised axial tomography may help. Treatment includes correction of hypoxia, hypercapnia and hypotension but in severely poisoned patients the latter may be extremely difficult until attempts are made to enhance the elimination of the poison. Hyperventilation of the patient till the Pa,co_2 lies between 3.0 and 3.4 kPa has been recommended for some forms of cerebral oedema but its feasibility and value in poisoned patients may be offset by coexisting severe hypotension. Mannitol 1 g/kg body weight in the form of a 20% solution should be given intravenously but for longer term management dexamethasone intramuscularly 10 mg followed by 4 mg 6-hourly is recommended, but it is not always effective in patients with generalised brain oedema. The patient should be nursed with the head elevated and fluid administration should be kept to the minimum.

Convulsions

Convulsions may complicate poisoning with many drugs, including CNS stimulants and anticholinergic compounds. If they are isolated and of brief duration, treatment is unnecessary but if frequently recurring or protracted they should be treated with intravenous diazepam. Patients who have a combination of vomiting and convulsions are at particular risk of inhalation of gastric contents. It may be safer to paralyse these patients and ventilate them mechanically until the poison has been metabolised and excreted.

Nerve and muscle compression injuries

Patients who lie unconscious in the same posture for long periods are in danger of nerve and muscle compression injuries. The nerves at particular risk are the radial, ulnar and lateral peroneal which lie relatively superficially and in relationship to bone. The damage is not usually evident until the patient regains consciousness and complains of numbness, paraesthesiae or weakness in the distribution of the nerve involved. Recovery is usually complete but may take several weeks or months.

Muscles subjected to protracted pressure frequently become necrotic and this may account for the elevation of serum enzyme levels known to occur in unconscious poisoned patients. Myoglobinuria leading to renal failure is an extremely rare sequel but myositis ossificans has been reported, particularly after poisoning with barbiturates and carbon monoxide. Extensive oedema and swelling within the confines of a fascial compartment may itself cause nerve or, rarely, arterial compression. In these cases the swelling is usually obvious and fasciotomy may be required.

Post-extubation laryngeal oedema

Some degree of laryngeal oedema probably occurs in every patient who has been intubated for more than a few hours but it seldom causes symptoms. In occasional cases, however, rebound hyperaemia of the cords with rapid accumulation of oedema may cause life-threatening laryngeal obstruction after extubation. It is particularly likely to develop in young women in whom the larynx tends to be relatively small and in whom the diameter of the endotracheal tube that can be accommodated is critical. Fluid overload, lying with the head down, and the chemical composition of the tube are also important aetiological factors.

Laryngeal oedema should be suspected when the patient develops stridor and signs of major airway obstruction within a few hours of extubation. Most settle when propped up to allow gravity to help reduce oedema and after being given warm, humidified, oxygen-enriched air by face mask. In severe cases tracheostomy may be necessary but should be avoided if at all possible, particularly in young women who will have to carry a prominent scar as a constant reminder of the episode for the rest of their lives.

Rare complications

Rare complications of acute poisoning include acute gastric dilatation and paralytic ileus. Respiratory tract burns may occur as a result of inhalation of hot, stimulant beverages administered to drowsy patients in well-intentioned, but futile, attempts to prevent them losing consciousness. Spinal artery thrombosis with consequent paraplegia rarely complicates prolonged, severe, hypotension.

THE RECOVERY PERIOD AND AFTER-CARE

Recovery

Disturbed behaviour

During recovery from overdoses of psychotropic drugs patients may exhibit grossly disturbed behaviour and can be a danger to themselves and others. This is commonly seen in association with anticholinergic compounds when patients frequently become agitated, delirious and hallucinated for two or three days. Large doses of diazepam may be required (p. 66).

Behaviour disturbance during recovery from barbiturate poisoning differs, particularly with phenobarbitone. The patient is usually disinhibited, loquacious, dysarthric, readily amused or, in some cases, aggressive and resentful of attention. In an unsupervised moment they may try to climb out of bed, often in a state of undress, and injure themselves. For their safety, to reduce subsequent embarrassment and for the peace of mind of relatives and staff, sedation is necessary. One dose of chlorpromazine (50 mg i.m.) is usually sufficient but some require more. This disinhibited state may be particularly prolonged and troublesome when phenobarbitone has been taken and in addition to sedation, forced alkaline diuresis may be indicated.

Psychiatric and social assessment

Following recovery from the physical effects of self-poisoning the patient should be interviewed to determine the cause for the episode and to identify any psychiatric illness or social precipitant which can be corrected. Whether this should be done by psychiatrists and social workers or by suitably trained general physicians is a matter of debate and will depend on the attitudes and enthusiasm of all concerned and the local availability of social and psychiatric services at short notice. Regardless of who accepts the role, it is essential that assessment is carried out as soon as possible after the overdose. Giving the patient an appointment to attend a psychiatric out-patient clinic at some time in the future is totally unsatisfactory because the default rate is so high.

Unfortunately, despite intensive psychiatric and social assessment, about 15–20 per cent of patients return within a year with another episode of self-poisoning, most occurring within three months of the first. The reasons are not difficult to identify:

1. Little can be done to reduce disagreement and violence between sexual partners and the reconciliation resulting from the first episode is often fragile and breaks down with little provocation. Advice to the partners to separate is often unrealistic since, in present-day society, tenancy of the home is usually in the man's name and the woman may have no refuge to which she can go.

2. Treatment for alcoholism, drug dependence and personality disorders is not nearly as successful as one would wish.

3. Psychiatric illness tends to relapse unpredictably.

4. The inherent nature of some of these individuals is such that they may create more of life's minor crises than the population as a whole and they are often less able to cope with them.

5. Involvement in crime is high among men who repeat self-poisoning and is not readily reduced.

6. Problems of substandard housing, high-rise living and unemployment require political rather than medical solutions.

7. The real patient may not be the individual who has taken the overdose but perhaps the violent, alcoholic husband who does not know, or will not accept, that he has a problem.

The clinician may not only predict and be unable to prevent the dissolution of many partnerships but, even more seriously, the inevitability of episodes of self-poisoning in any offspring. Self-poisoning in teenagers is frequently associated with conflict with parents, truancy, failure to attain academic performance compatible with intelligence, early experimentation with drugs and alcohol and involvement in petty crime. These are the most depressing and disturbing facets of self-poisoning but when one considers the incidence of precipitating factors in the population it becomes surprising that the repeat rate is so low. Many people must come to terms with what others would consider to be an appalling environment and they deserve sympathy, understanding and help. Government at all levels must also help find solutions to some of the problems.

Review of regular drug treatment

General considerations

Following recovery from an episode of self-poisoning, the opportunity should be taken to review the patient's regular drug treatment. Despite the average age, many are on regular treatment, particularly with psychotropic drugs which they may have been taking for weeks, months or even years. It is commonplace to meet patients who have been taking two or three different types of psychotropic drug concurrently (e.g. a tranquilliser, antidepressant and hypnotic). It must also be remembered that about 60 per cent of patients who take drug overdoses do so with medicines which they have been prescribed and another 15 per cent take drugs which have been prescribed for close relatives. Rationalisation of prescribing may help reduce morbidity related to regular drug ingestion and also diminish the availability of drugs for repeated episodes of self-poisoning.

Benzodiazepines

Undoubtedly benzodiazepines are the most widely used and appear to be prescribed indiscriminately for young and middle-aged women who are unduly anxious, have marital problems, difficulty in coping with children and a variety of other social stresses. Clearly drugs cannot resolve these problems but may blunt the individual's response to them and make them more tolerable. On the other hand, it is possible that some patients become so drugged that they are even less capable of coping than they were in the first place. When questioned, some patients spontaneously admit that tranquillisers were unhelpful or made them even more depressed. It has also been suggested that benzodiazepines, like alcohol, release aggression and fuel the inter-personal conflict which so commonly precedes self-poisoning. Commonly, one meets patients who have been prescribed two and occasionally three different benzodiazepines presumably in the mistaken belief that their actions are radically different. Psychiatric patients in particular are likely to get into difficulties if drugs are prescribed by the hospital and by the family doctor concurrently.

Analgesics

Analgesics are another group of drugs which may be prescribed for long periods and have effects on cerebral function. This is particularly true of the narcotic analgesics, dextropropoxyphene, dihydrocodeine and dipipanone, especially if prescribed in conjunction with tranquillisers, antidepressants, hypnotics or anticonvulsants.

On other occasions patients may be taking drugs with contrary actions on the central nervous system (e.g. appetite suppressants which stimulate the brain and benzodiazepines or hypnotics which depress it, ergotamine preparations for migraine and vasodilators because of cold hands, phenothiazines and anticholinergic drugs, depressants and antidepressants). There is considerable scope for the rationalisation of drug treatment or even the discontinuation of some drugs in most patients.

Advice about driving

Recovery from minor overdoses of psychotropic drugs appears to take place very quickly and the patient is soon able to walk steadily, talk coherently and to be interviewed. This may lull the physician into thinking that the effects of the drugs have disappeared completely before the patient is discharged. However, this is not the case and many drugs, most importantly the benzodiazepines, have persistent active metabolites, which will continue to act on the brain for several days or weeks after the overdose. These may be sufficient to impair co-ordination and reflexes and therefore the ability to perform complex tasks such as driving a motor vehicle or operating complicated machinery with safety. The doctor clearly has a responsibility to the general public as well as to the individual recovering from the drug overdose. The patient must be warned against participating in such activities for a variable period of time, the length of which has to be judged from a knowledge of the drugs involved in individual cases. It must also be stressed to the patient that the effects of alcohol will be potentiated during this time.

POINTS OF EMPHASIS

- All but a small minority of unconscious poisoned patients recover with supportive care alone.

- A clear airway is imperative.

- Improving the airway alone may improve ventilation, hypotension and level of consciousness.

- Arterial blood gas analysis is essential for the assessment of ventilation.

- Arterial hydrogen ion concentrations and oxygen and carbon dioxide tensions should be corrected for body temperature.

- Hypotension usually responds to simple measures to increase venous return.

- Correct hypercapnia before correcting metabolic acidosis.

- Consult the poisons information services if you are in doubt about the constituents, toxicity or treatment of poisoning with any product.

- Speak personally to a physician at the poisons information service if there is difficulty.

- Antidotes, particularly for narcotic analgesics, paracetamol and iron salts, may be life-saving.

- Induced emesis using syrup of ipecacuanha is the method of choice for emptying the stomach in conscious children.

- Never use salt solution as an emetic.

- Never attempt gastric emptying by any method if the airway cannot be protected.

- Emergency drug analyses are only indicated if the result will alter management.

- Measurement of plasma drug concentrations is mandatory before attempting forced diuresis, haemodialysis and haemoperfusion to eliminate drugs.

- Humidify and warm the inspired air for patients with endotracheal tubes.

- Manage skin blisters as burns.

- The eyes of unconscious patients must be kept lubricated and closed to avoid exposure damage.

- Unconscious poisoned patients seldom require more than 2.0 litres of intravenous fluid daily.

- Indiscriminate catheterisation of every unconscious patient is unacceptable.

- Hypothermia does not require rapid correction or heroic treatment.

- Forced alkaline diuresis is the method of choice for enhancing elimination of salicylates and phenobarbitone.

- Charcoal or resin haemoperfusion should be used to eliminate CNS depressants—but only in very severe poisoning.

- Pulmonary oedema complicating acute poisoning is often the result of misguided attempts to force a diuresis.

- Renal failure should be treated conventionally.

- Cerebral oedema should be anticipated in patients who have had prolonged hypotension or cardio-respiratory arrest.

- Disturbed behaviour is common during recovery.

- Every patient who has deliberately poisoned himself must be assessed to identify correctable psychiatric and social precipitants.

- Review the patient's drug treatment after self-poisoning.

- Advise the patient about driving and other complex tasks after overdosage with psychotropic drugs.

CHAPTER 4

Features and treatment of specific poisons

ACETONE

General considerations

Acetone is a volatile and inflammable organic solvent widely used in laboratories and domestically for nail varnish removal. It is one of the solvents abused by 'glue sniffers' and can be absorbed through the lungs, skin and alimentary tract. Serious poisoning with acetone is rare.

Features

Depression of consciousness and respiration are the most serious consequences. The breath smells of acetone and the throat may be inflamed, oedematous and show superficial ulceration if the acetone has been taken internally. Glycosuria and hyperglycaemia have been reported and the oral glucose tolerance curve may be diabetic in character. The mechanism of glucose intolerance is not known. Acetone will be present in the urine. Liver function is not disturbed.

Treatment

The patient should be removed from the toxic atmosphere and contaminated clothing must be removed and the skin thoroughly washed. The stomach should be emptied if the acetone was ingested within the preceding 4 hours. Supportive measures will be required if the patient is unconscious but there is no specific treatment. Hyperglycaemia may require control with insulin.

Prognosis

Recovery of consciousness may be anticipated within a few hours. Glucose tolerance may take a few months to return to normal.

Reference

Gitelson S, Werczberger A, Herman JB. Coma and hyperglycaemia following drinking of acetone. *Diabetes* 1966; **15**: 810–811.

ADDER ENVENOMATION

General considerations

The adder, *Vipera berus*, is found widely throughout Western Europe and is the only naturally occurring poisonous snake in the United Kingdom. Bites usually result from trying to pick up the snake but may also occur if it is taken unawares. They are only likely to be encountered in the summer months since the adder hibernates during the winter. Probably less than 50 per cent of bites are associated with the injection of venom.

Features

The bite comprises two puncture marks about a centimetre apart and usually occurs on the extremity of a limb. It may go unnoticed apart from swelling but more often there is immediate pain. Swelling at the site is usually apparent within an hour and is a certain indicator of the injection of venom. However, systemic poisoning may occur in the absence of local reaction. Vomiting, abdominal pain and diarrhoea may occur within a few minutes and occasionally transient shock and loss of consciousness also occur at a very early stage. Gastrointestinal symptoms may continue for two days and over this time the limb swelling extends and becomes haemorrhagic. In the worst cases the trunk, face and lips may become swollen. Shock may persist or occur up to 36 hours after the bite and this together with development of bleeding, oliguria, a neutrophil leukocytosis and non-specific ECG changes indicates severe systemic poisoning.

Investigation and monitoring

The pulse rate and blood pressure should be recorded hourly for 48 hours and a careful note should be made of the urinary output and the volumes of fluid lost through vomiting and diarrhoea. The extent of swelling should be recorded daily and the girth of the proximal and distal parts of the limb should be measured about the mid-points.

The white cell count, plasma urea and electrolytes should be measured daily. An ECG should be performed twice daily or the cardiac rhythm monitored continuously if hypotension is present. A coagulation screen is indicated if bleeding occurs.

Treatment

Reassurance of the victim is one of the most important aspects of first aid. The bite should not be incised or sucked but cleaned and covered with a dry dressing. If hospital is more than 30 minutes away a bandage or light ligature should be placed round the limb proximal to the bite and should be tight enough to impede venous return without obstructing arterial inflow. If practicable the limb should not be used since muscle activity will facilitate absorption of venom from the bite. The affected limb should be kept dependent.

Every victim should be referred to hospital and observed for at least 24 hours. Remove any ligature that is present. Symptomatic treatment may be required for undue anxiety, pain or vomiting but antibiotics, corticosteroids and anti-tetanus treatment are unnecessary. Local application of ice-packs may add to tissue necrosis and should not be used.

The only antivenom of value is the Zagreb antivenom. The principal indications for its use are persistent or recurrent hypotension, bleeding, ECG changes and leukocytosis ($>20\,000/mm^3$). Administration of antivenom should also be considered in adults in whom swelling has extended up the limb within two hours of the bite to reduce disability from the local effects of the poison. Two ampoules of the antivenom (the dose does not vary with age) should be added to 100 ml normal saline and infused at a rate of fifteen drops/minute. The benefits of antivenom have to be weighed against the risk of hypersensitivity reactions to the serum. A history of asthma or other allergic condition is therefore a relative contraindication to its use. The subcutaneous injection of a small dose as a test of serum hypersensitivity is of no value and may give misleading results. Immediate reactions to antivenom can be satisfactorily controlled by temporarily stopping the infusion and prompt intramuscular injection of 0.5 ml of 1:1000 adrenaline which *must* be drawn into the syringe *before* giving antivenom.

Prognosis

Death from adder envenomation is extremely rare and many more deaths have been reported from bee and wasp stings.

Patients under the age of 14 years usually recover completely in three weeks or less while many adults take significantly longer.

References

Reid HA. Adder bites in Britain. *Br Med J* 1976; **2**: 153–156.
Theakston RDG, Reid HA. Effectiveness of Zagreb antivenom against envenomation by the adder, *Vipera berus. Lancet* 1976; **2**: 121–123.

AMPHETAMINES AND RELATED DRUGS

Amphetamines	*Chemically related drugs*
Amphetamine	Diethylpropion
Dexamphetamine	Fencamfamin
Methylamphetamine	Fenfluramine
	Methylphenidate
	Phenmetrazine
	Phentermine

General considerations

Acute poisoning with amphetamines and chemically related anorectic and stimulant drugs occurs fairly frequently but is seldom serious. Poisoning may be the result of an acute overdose or may be due to longer-term increasing doses taken by addicts. Amphetamines are frequently formulated in combination with barbiturates and when overdoses of such preparations are taken it is usually the amphetamine toxicity which predominates.

Features

The major features of amphetamine intoxication result from CNS stimulation and sympathomimetic actions. Early signs include talkativeness, restlessness, tachycardia, tachypnoea, tremor and dilated pupils. Facial flushing and sweating may also be present and as poisoning becomes worse confusion, delirium, hallucinations, paranoia and violence towards himself and others become prominent. The blood pressure may rise to extreme levels leading to intracerebral, subarachnoid and subdural haemorrhage and brain stem petechiae. Cardiac dysrhythmias, particularly ventricular fibrillation, hyperpyrexia and convulsions may be fatal.

Treatment

The stomach should be emptied if more than fifteen tablets have been taken within the preceding 4 hours.

Haloperidol (5–10 mg) and droperidol (5–15 mg) are the most effective drugs for counteracting the central effects of amphetamines and should be given slowly intravenously, titrating the dose against the clinical response. Chlorpromazine is less effective but may be used if droperidol is not available. Barbiturates are of less value.

When poisoning is severe urinary excretion of amphetamines may be enhanced by inducing a forced acid diuresis (p. 46) provided the appropriate precautions are observed.

Hyperpyrexia and convulsions should be treated symptomatically. Extreme tachycardia will respond to β-adrenergic blockers but cardiac dysrhythmias should not be treated unless life-threatening, prolonged or recurring frequently.

References

Gary NE, Saidi P. Methamphetamine intoxication. A speedy new treatment. *Am J Med* 1978; **64**: 537–539.

von Mühlendahl KE, Krienke EG. Fenfluramine poisoning. *Clin Toxicol* 1979; **14**: 97–106.

Rappolt RT, Gay GR. Treatment plan for acute and chronic adrenergic poisoning crises utilising sympatholytic effects of the B^1–B^2 receptor site blocker propranolol (Inderal) in concert with diazepam and urine acidification. *Clin Toxicol* 1979; **14**: 55–69.

ANTIBIOTICS

General considerations

Despite the wide availability of antibiotics in the community it is uncommon to encounter individuals who have poisoned themselves with these drugs. With the exception of anti-tuberculosis drugs (considered separately), antibiotics are remarkably non-toxic in overdosage.

Features

The majority of patients will have no ill-effects. Occasionally transient nausea, vomiting and diarrhoea may occur.

Treatment

No specific treatment is required. Gastrointestinal upsets should be treated symptomatically if severe or prolonged. A good fluid intake should be encouraged.

ANTICHOLINERGIC COMPOUNDS

Anti-diarrhoeal drugs
Atropine
Propantheline

Antihistamines
Chlorpheniramine
Diphenhydramine
Methapyrilene
Promethazine
Trimeprazine

Anti-parkinsonian drugs
Amantidine
Benzhexol
Benztropine
Orphenadrine
Procyclidine

Mydriatic eye drops
Atropine
Cyclopentolate
Homatropine

Plants
Atropa belladonna
Datura species (arborea, candida, metel, rosei, stramonium, suaveolens)

Tetracyclic antidepressant
Maprotiline

Tricyclic antidepressants
Amitriptyline
Dothiepin
Doxepin
Imipramine
Nortriptyline
Protriptyline
Trimipramine

General considerations

These compounds comprise one of the most important groups of poisons encountered in clinical practice. They are grouped together because many of the features of poisoning are due to an anticholinergic action but they also have significant quinidine-like effects. Tricyclic antidepressants are particularly important since they are taken by about 13 per cent of adults who poison themselves and they are also prescribed for enuretic children who may accidentally take them in overdosage. Some pleasantly-flavoured cough mixtures contain antihistamines and may be taken by young children who may also be attracted by the shiny black berries of *Atropa belladonna,* the deadly nightshade. Teenagers and young adults occasionally take anti-parkinsonian drugs or concoctions of parts of plants of the *Datura* species for 'kicks' (especially *Datura stramonium,* the Jimson weed, and *Datura suaveolens,* angel's trumpet). Extracts of *Datura stramonium* are also contained in some herbal asthma remedies (Asthmador powder, Potter's asthma powder and Surama cigarettes) which are virtually harmless if smoked but toxic if taken orally.

Features

Effects of anticholinergic drugs are peripheral, cardiac and central.

1. *Peripheral effects* include warm, dry skin due to vasodilation and inhibition of sweating, blurring of vision from paralysis of accommodation and pupillary dilatation and urinary retention. Hypotension due to anticholinergic compounds is less frequent than with barbiturate poisoning causing comparable depression of consciousness.

2. *Cardiac effects* of anticholinergic drugs have received considerable attention but, apart from sinus tachycardia due to vagal blockade which occurs in over half the cases, they are by no means as common as the literature might suggest. The incidence of the major effects of tricyclic antidepressants are given in Table 4.1.

Prolongation of the PR interval and widening of the QRS complex occur commonly and when the P wave is lost in the preceding T wave the changes are often mistakenly diagnosed as a ventricular dysrhythmia. Supraventricular and ventricular dysrhythmias do occur in a very small minority of patients and may be the cause of

TABLE 4.1   Incidence of anticholinergic effects in 219 consecutive cases of poisoning with tricyclic antidepressants.

Feature	Conscious patients (%) (n = 135)	Unconscious patients* (%) (n = 84)	All patients (%) (n = 219)
Strabismus	18	81	42
Urinary retention	18	65	36
Convulsions	1	10	4
Sinus tachycardia			
100–119/min	37	68	49
120/min	8	13	10
Conduction defects and			
dysrhythmias	0	12	4
Delirium and			
hallucinations	10	35	19

*Coma grades 2, 3 and 4.

sudden deaths shortly after ingestion of the overdose. Paradoxically, a bradycardia is present in some cases. Deaths have been reported to occur up to several days after apparent recovery from poisoning. During the recovery phase the cardiac effects disappear in reverse order, usually within 12–24 hours.

3. *Central effects* include coma, respiratory depression and hypothermia. Coma is more commonly grade 2 or 3 than grade 4 and the lighter grades are associated with divergent strabismus, increased muscle tone, myoclonus, hyperreflexia, and extensor plantar responses. However, in very deep coma these features may be absent and it may be impossible to elicit plantar reflexes. Convulsions occur in a small proportion of cases during the early stages of intoxication but they are usually of short duration.

Delirium and hallucinations may be present briefly before coma supervenes but are commoner during recovery. The patient is usually restless, continuously plucking at the bedclothes and muttering to some relative who is not present. There is often considerable dysarthria, partly due to dryness of the mouth and tongue, and speech is extremely rapid, often of low volume and incomprehensible. These features are normally accompanied by jerky, semi-purposive movements of the eyes, head, limbs and trunk as if the patient is constantly being distracted by events in the environment, each competing for attention. The hallucinations are predominantly visual, taking the form of familiar people or objects, and are not usually as distressing as those of delirium tremens. The patient usually has complete amnesia for these events which may persist uninterrupted by sleep or sedation for two to three days. In some cases, however, the hallucinations are clearly frightening or there may be complete recall on recovery.

Plasma concentrations of tricyclic antidepressants

Plasma concentrations of tricyclic antidepressants cannot be measured readily in hospital laboratories. Limited studies in children showed that plasma concentrations below 500 μg/l are associated with anticholinergic features but not cardiac dysrhythmias or convulsions, whereas the latter tend to occur with concentrations above 1000 μg/l. Similarly plasma concentrations correlate fairly well with severity of toxicity in adults. Elevation of plasma drug levels may be prolonged and explain the late toxic effects. Knowledge of plasma concentrations does not alter management and is unnecessary in the emergency situation.

Treatment

General measures

The stomach should be emptied if more than 15 tablets have been taken within four hours of admission or if the patient is unconscious. Coma should be managed in the conventional way paying particular attention to the adequacy of ventilation. Cardiac monitoring should be carried out in unconscious patients.

Convulsions

Convulsions are usually short-lived and infrequent. They often do not require treatment but if prolonged or recurring at short intervals, they may be controlled with intravenous diazepam. It is important to avoid unnecessary stimulation of the patient.

Delirium and hallucinations

Treatment of delirium and hallucinations may be necessary to alleviate distress and to reduce overactivity so that the patient does not cause self injury. Diazepam orally is adequate but large doses (up to 50 mg hourly) may be required initially to achieve the desired effect. Further doses are given according to the patient's condition.

Urinary retention

It is usually possible to empty a distended bladder by applying suprapubic pressure and catheterisation should be avoided unless this is unsuccessful.

Cardiac dysrhythmias

The treatment of cardiac conduction abnormalities and dysrhythmias is controversial. Their aetiology is poorly understood and many doctors unrealistically expect them to respond to drugs used for similar problems complicating myocardial infarction. Anti-arrhythmic drugs are themselves cardiac poisons and their indiscriminate use merely adds to the toxicological confusion. Conduction defects and dysrhythmias due to anticholinergic compounds should not be 'treated' provided the patient is perfusing tissues adequately and is maintaining an acceptable blood pressure. In difficult cases with circulatory failure, physostigmine salicylate or anti-arrhythmic therapy (usually β-adrenergic blockers or lignocaine) may have to be given on a trial and error basis. Sometimes it may be impossible to decide the true nature of serious anticholinergic drug dysrhythmias and in these cases His bundle electrocardiography may be of diagnostic help and also be of value in monitoring the effects of treatment. It has been suggested that the toxicity of tricyclic antidepressants may be reduced by rapid intravenous infusion of sodium bicarbonate (1–3 mmol/kg over 20 min) and this should be tried before resorting to anti-arrhythmic drugs.

Physostigmine salicylate

The toxic effects of anticholinergic drugs can be reversed by cholinesterase inhibitors such as physostigmine salicylate, a tertiary ammonium compound which is able to cross the blood–brain barrier. It is usually given in a dose of 2 mg intravenously over 2 minutes for an adult or 0.5 mg for a child and within 5–10 minutes the heart rate slows and, depending on the initial depth of coma, consciousness may be regained or coma become less deep. Delirious, hallucinating patients given physostigmine rapidly become rational and lucid. Unfortunately physostigmine is metabolised rapidly and its effects last no more than 30 minutes. This disadvantage could be overcome by giving repeated boluses or a constant infusion but there are other drawbacks to its use. It may precipitate convulsions, cause a troublesome increase in salivation and bronchial secretions and has been reported to cause ventricular tachycardia. More importantly, there is no evidence that treatment with physostigmine is superior to supportive management and its role in the treatment of dysrhythmias is uncertain. Administration of physostigmine may be used as a diagnostic test for anticholinergic poisoning in cases where the cause of coma is in doubt. Its use is also justifiable in unconscious patients with serious respiratory complications in whom an early return of consciousness is desirable.

Measures to increase elimination

Tricyclic antidepressants have a very large volume of distribution and are eliminated by hepatic metabolism. As a consequence, forced diuresis and peritoneal and haemodialysis are of no value in the treatment of poisoning. Limited experience with charcoal and resin haemoperfusion suggests that this technique is ineffective.

Prognosis

The outlook for patients who reach medical care is excellent. Unconscious patients generally show significant improvement within 12 hours and regain consciousness within 36 hours. Cardiac conduction abnormalities and dysrhythmias usually resolve within 12 hours but delirium and hallucinations may persist for 2–3 days or even longer.

References

Aquilonius S-M, Hedstrand U. The use of physostigmine as an antidote in tricyclic antidepressant intoxication. *Acta Anaesthesiol Scand* 1978; **22**: 40–45.

Barnett AH, Jones FW, Williams ER. Acute poisoning with Potter's asthma remedy. *Br Med J* 1977; **2**: 1635.

Belton PA, Gibbons DO. Datura intoxication in West Cornwall. *Br Med J* 1979; **1**: 585–586.

Bobik A, McLean AJ. Cardiovascular complications due to pheniramine overdosage. *Aust NZ J Med* 1976; **6**: 65–67.

Cowen PJ. Toxic psychosis with antihistamines reversed by physostigmine. *Postgrad Med J* 1979; **55**: 556–557.

Crome P, Newman B. The problem of tricyclic antidepressant poisoning. *Postgrad Med J* 1979; **55**: 528–532.

Hershey LA. The use and abuse of physostigmine. *Drug Therapy* 1980; **10**: 143–148.

Hestand HE, Teske DW. Diphenhydramine hydrochloride intoxication. *J Pediatr* 1979; **90**: 1017–1018.

Levy R. Arrhythmias following physostigmine administration in Jimson weed poisoning. *J A C E P* 1977; **6**: 107–108.

Nattel S, Bayne L, Ruedy J. Physostigmine in coma due to drug overdose. *Clin Pharmacol Ther* 1979; **25**: 96–102.

Park J, Proudfoot AT. Acute poisoning with maprotiline hydrochloride. *Br Med J* 1977; **1**: 1573.

Shervette RE, Schydlower M, Lampe RM, Fearnow RG. Jimson 'loco' weed abuse in adolescents. *Pediatrics* 1979; **63**: 520–523.

Starkey IR, Lawson AAH. Poisoning with tricyclic and related antidepressants—a ten year review. *Q J Med* 1980; New Series **49**: 33–49.

BARBITURATES

Amylobarbitone	Phenobarbitone
Butobarbitone	Quinalbarbitone
Cyclobarbitone	Sodium amylobarbitone
Pentobarbitone	

General considerations

During the 1960's barbiturates were the most common drugs taken in overdosage and were responsible for a major proportion of poisoning deaths. Since then their role as hypnotics and sedatives has been largely supplanted by the benzodiazepines, and barbiturate overdosage now comprises no more than 10 per cent of U.K. hospital admissions for self-poisoning. It can be expected that this form of poisoning will continue to become less common though phenobarbitone poisoning will probably remain a problem because of its widespread use as an anticonvulsant. Barbiturates are also greatly abused, not only by addicts who take large quantities by mouth or by mainlining, but also by enormous numbers of middle-aged and elderly women who have become physically and psychologically dependent on them after many years of use for night sedation.

The former classification of barbiturates into short-, medium- and long-acting groups is inappropriate and misleading. The duration of coma after overdosage is comparable for all the barbiturates except phenobarbitone. This has a much longer duration of action which, together with other properties, is sufficiently important for it to be considered separately (see p. 175). By far the most common barbiturate preparation taken in overdosage or by addicts is a combination of quinalbarbitone and sodium amylobarbitone (Tuinal).

Features

The principal features of barbiturate poisoning result from generalised CNS depression. Drowsiness, ataxia and dysarthria are soon followed by coma, hypotension, respiratory depression and hypothermia. Barbiturates were formerly responsible for about half the cases of deep coma (grades 3 and 4) after poisoning, and though their contribution is decreasing, it is still important. As coma deepens, the gag and cough reflexes disappear and breathing becomes shallow though the respiratory rate remains normal or only slightly reduced. The pupils are neither constricted nor dilated but the limbs become hypotonic with loss of tendon reflexes. The plantar response, if present, is flexor but in deep coma may be absent. In about six per cent of patients with barbiturate poisoning the skin over pressure areas becomes erythematous, oedematous and goes on to blister (p. 15) but non-pressure areas (e.g. interdigital clefts) may develop similar lesions. These changes are probably the result of a combination of pressure and a direct toxic effect on the epidermis. Addicts who have been injecting barbiturates intravenously will show the usual hallmarks of repeated injections and may have indolent necrotic skin ulcers where the irritant drug solution has leaked into the subcutaneous tissues.

Plasma barbiturate concentrations

Most clinical chemistry laboratories measure plasma barbiturate concentrations on an emergency basis but the results frequently have to be interpreted with caution because some analytical methods in common use measure inactive metabolites in addition to unchanged drug.

In general, plasma concentrations correlate rather poorly with the depth of coma partly because of tolerance to the drugs and partly because of simultaneous ingestion of other CNS depressants, including ethanol. However, for any given grade of coma the plasma concentrations of cyclobarbitone and butobarbitone tend to be higher than those of amylobarbitone, pentobarbitone and quinalbarbitone. Concentrations after overdosage decline slowly initially, then more rapidly as enzyme induction develops acutely. Many texts refer to 'fatal' plasma barbiturate concentrations but it is not uncommon to encounter patients who are drug tolerant awake and talking with plasma barbiturate concentrations well into the so-called lethal range.

Emergency measurement of plasma barbiturate concentrations is commonly requested but is seldom justified since the result rarely alters management.

Treatment

The stomach should be emptied if more than fifteen tablets or capsules have been taken in the preceding 4 hours or if the patient is unconscious. Coma is managed conventionally (p. 24) and skin bullae as outlined on p. 42.

The axiom that treatment should be determined by the patient's clinical state rather than the plasma drug concentration was never more true than in poisoning with barbiturate hypnotics. All but a small minority of those who reach hospital survive with careful, undramatic support of vital functions alone. Forced diuresis, peritoneal dialysis and haemodialysis intended to increase elimination of barbiturates from the body are potentially hazardous and largely inefficient. Those patients who are desperately ill, in deep coma with severe hypotension, respiratory complications, or who deteriorate or fail to improve despite intensive care should be treated by charcoal haemoperfusion. At present this is the method of choice for increasing elimination of barbiturates from the body but only patients satisfying the criteria on p. 49 should be treated in this way.

Prognosis

The great majority of deaths from barbiturate poisoning occur outside hospital and before medical care is possible. It is widely stated that the hospital mortality is less than one per cent but most surveys claiming this degree of success include many patients with mild intoxication who were never at risk in the first place. The mortality increases with increasing depth of coma and is probably of the order of 5 per cent in grade 4 coma despite high standards of supportive care. Death usually results from shock, cerebral oedema and respiratory infections.

References

Bismuth C, Conso F, Wattel F, et al. Coated activated charcoal hemoperfusion. *Vet Human Toxicol* 1979; **21**: 81–83.

Dymock RB, James RA, Lokan RJ. Tuinal as a drug of abuse. *Med J Aust* 1980; **2**: 214–215.

Goodman JM, Bischel MD, Wagers PW, Barbour BH. Barbiturate intoxication. *West J Med* 1976; **124**: 179–186.

Greenblatt DJ, Allen MD, Harmatz JS, Noel BJ, Shader RI. Overdosage with pentobarbital and secobarbital: assessment of factors related to outcome. *J Clin Pharmacol* 1979; **19**: 758–768.

Iversen BM, Willassen Y, Bakke OM, Wallem G. Assessment of barbiturate removal by charcoal hemoperfusion in overdose cases. *Clin Toxicol* 1979; **15**: 139–149.

Koffler A, Bernstein M, LaSette A, Massry SG. Fixed-bed charcoal hemoperfusion. *Arch Intern Med* 1978; **138**: 1691–1694.

Matthew H. Barbiturates. *Clin Toxicol* 1975; **8**: 495–513.

BENZENE HEXACHLORIDE

General considerations

Gamma benzene hexachloride (hexachlorocyclohexane) is an insecticide widely used for the treatment of scabies and pediculosis. It is readily and rapidly absorbed from the gastro-intestinal tract and is highly lipid-soluble. Acute poisoning is uncommon but more frequent in children.

Features

Consciousness is rapidly lost and myoclonus and convulsions may occur. Muscle tone is greatly increased and the reflexes are exaggerated. Vomiting is common and constantly threatens the airway. Renal tubular and hepatocellular necrosis, severe acidaemia, delayed pancreatitis and proximal myopathy with myoglobinuria have been reported.

A polymorph leukocytosis is commonly found and serum aspartate aminotransferase and lactic dehydrogenase activity may be increased.

Treatment

There is no specific treatment for this type of poisoning. The stomach should be emptied if the poison has been taken within four hours and after taking appropriate steps to safeguard the airway. Arterial blood gas analysis should be carried out and any acid-base abnormality corrected. The combination of coma, vomiting and convulsions is particularly dangerous. Isolated convulsions do not require treatment but if frequent, control is best obtained by curarisation and mechanical ventilation rather than by attempts to suppress fits with intravenous diazepam. Other problems are treated symptomatically as they arise.

Prognosis

Benzene hexachloride is rapidly metabolised and redistributed in adipose tissue. Recovery of consciousness can be expected within about 12 hours. Convulsions subside during this time but the patient may remain drowsy and irritable for 24–48 hours. Once consciousness is regained survival is likely.

References

Munk ZM, Nantel A. Acute lindane poisoning with development of muscle necrosis. *Can Med Assoc J* 1977; **117**: 1050–1054.
Wheeler M. Gamma benzene hydrochloride (Kwell) poisoning in a child. *West J Med* 1977; **127**: 518–521.

BENZODIAZEPINES

Chlorazepate	Flurazepam	Oxazepam
Chlordiazepoxide	Lorazepam	Temazepam
Clonazepam	Medazepam	Triazolam
Diazepam	Nitrazepam	

General considerations

The benzodiazepines were introduced in the early 1960's and have since been prescribed on an increasing scale. They are now involved in about 40 per cent of drug overdoses in the U.K. Although benzodiazepines in overdosage have a remarkable and unique degree of safety they can potentiate the toxicity of other CNS depressants taken simultaneously. The use of benzodiazepines, and consequently benzodiazepine poisoning, is more common among women than men probably because they are socially more acceptable than alcohol, which is the 'tranquilliser' preferred by men.

Features

Benzodiazepines taken alone

All benzodiazepines produce similar effects. When taken alone, they cause drowsiness, apathy, ataxia, dysarthria, partial ptosis and nystagmus. Coma, seldom deeper than grade 2, may follow. There may be mild hypotension and respiratory depression. Though they have been shown to exacerbate hypoxia and hypercapnia in patients with chronic obstructive airways disease, this rarely causes serious problems.

Bullous skin lesions have been reported after overdosage with nitrazepam. Some patients, particularly the elderly, show increased susceptibility to the toxic effects of benzodiazepines but in general large quantities (commonly up to 0.5 g diazepam or 0.8 g chlordiazepoxide) can be taken without causing serious illness and uncomplicated recovery has been reported after ingestion of 2 g diazepam, 1.15 g chlordiazepoxide and 2.4 g oxazepam. Though unsubstantiated, clinical impression suggests that flurazepam (or more probably its major active metabolite) causes deeper and longer-lasting CNS depression than comparable overdoses of other benzodiazepines. The great majority of patients poisoned with benzodiazepines alone recover considerably within 24 hours. It must be remembered that many benzodiazepines have active metabolites with long plasma half-lives so that performance in skilled tasks (e.g. driving motor vehicles) may be impaired for several days or weeks after apparent recovery from the overdose and patients should be warned accordingly.

Benzodiazepines with other drugs

Benzodiazepines are commonly taken in overdosage with other psychotropic drugs and potentiate the CNS depressant effects of barbiturates, ethanol and tricyclic antidepressants. Their combination with the last named has advantages since their anticonvulsant properties may prevent convulsions from the anticholinergic drugs and they also help to control the delirium and hallucinations.

Though deaths from CNS depression have been attributed to benzodiazepine overdosage alone, clinical experience suggests that this is highly improbable and the fatal cases have seldom been sufficiently well studied to exclude the possibility that death was due to other drugs.

Treatment

The toxic effects of benzodiazepines taken alone are so minimal that little treatment is required. Emptying the stomach is probably valueless unless more than 30 tablets or capsules have been taken within 4 hours. Impairment of consciousness and hypotension should be treated conventionally (p. 24).

References

Finkle BS, McCloskey KL, Goodman LS. Diazepam and drug-associated deaths. *JAMA* 1979; **242**: 429–434.
Greenblatt DJ, Woo E, Allen MD, Orsulak PJ, Shader RI. Rapid recovery from massive diazepam overdose. *JAMA* 1978; **240**: 1872–1874.
Solomon K. Safety of oxazepam. *NY State J Med* 1978; **78**: 91–92.

BETA-ADRENERGIC BLOCKING DRUGS

Atenolol	Practolol
Metoprolol	Propranolol
Oxprenolol	Sotalol

General considerations

Acute overdosage with beta-adrenergic blocking drugs has been reported relatively infrequently considering their current widespread use for treatment of hypertension, dysrhythmias and angina pectoris. Though this group of drugs contains many members only the few listed above have to date been involved in poisoning episodes. Almost certainly the others will have similar effects.

Features

There is controversy about the toxicity of large overdoses of beta-adrenergic blockers. While some patients have apparently ingested massive doses without ill effects the majority of reports indicate life-threatening consequences even in those with normal cardiovascular systems.

The onset of symptoms may be unexpectedly rapid. Pallor and ataxia progress to coma with peripheral circulatory failure and cold, clammy, cyanosed extremities. Profound bradycardia is usually present with a reduced or unrecordable blood pressure. Convulsions, respiratory arrest or asystolic cardiac arrest may occur at any moment.

Electrocardiograms may show that the bradycardia is sinus in origin but it may be very difficult to identify P waves with certainty. There may be marked QRS prolongation and ST and T wave changes. The plasma potassium may be raised.

Treatment

The stomach should be emptied as speedily as possible. Severe bradycardia and hypotension may respond to atropine 3 mg intravenously (or 0.04 mg/kg) which may be repeated if necessary. The heart rate and rhythm should be monitored continuously.

If atropine is ineffective an isoprenaline infusion may set up and the rate of administration increased until the desired increase in pulse rate and blood pressure is achieved. Since the isoprenaline is in competition with the beta-blocker at receptor sites very large amounts may have to be given. Failure to appreciate this may account for the early reports of isoprenaline 'resistance' in beta-blocker poisoning.

Glucagon is a useful and apparently safe alternative to isoprenaline and is the treatment of choice. It is thought to work by activating adenylcyclase by a mechanism which is not blocked by beta-blockers. A single bolus of 5–10 mg has dramatic effects on the pulse and blood pressure and vomiting may be induced. In severe poisoning the response to glucagon may be transient and an infusion of 4 mg/h should be given and reduced gradually as the patient improves. When large quantities have to be given it is preferable to use a preparation of glucagon which does not contain phenol as a preservative, or to use 5% dextrose instead of the diluent provided.

Convulsions should not be treated if they are short-lived and infrequent.

Reference

Leading Article. Beta-blocker poisoning. *Lancet* 1980; **1**: 803–804.

BLEACHES

General considerations

The active constituent of most household bleaches is sodium hypochlorite in concentrations up to 10 per cent. Bleaches have a corrosive action due partly to the alkalinity of the solution and partly to the formation of hypochlorous acid and liberation of free chlorine when hypochlorite reacts with gastric acid. The chlorine may, in turn, be inhaled and cause respiratory symptoms. Poisoning with household bleaches is largely confined to children below the age of five years.

Features

The majority of children who accidentally ingest bleach presumably take only small quantities and do not develop symptoms. About 35 per cent have nausea and/or vomiting and 20 per cent irritation of the buccal mucosa. Ulceration of mucous membranes and abdominal pain are uncommon. In contrast, the deliberate ingestion of large quantities can be fatal due to oesophageal ulceration, perforation, haemorrhage and shock. Cough and laryngeal oedema may develop if free chlorine is inhaled.

Treatment

Very little treatment is required for most patients. If only small amounts have been ingested it will be sufficient to give milk or antacids. The stomach should be emptied if a large quantity has been taken and (if readily available) sodium thiosulphate left in the stomach to reduce any remaining hypochlorite. Severe poisoning with corrosive oesophagitis or gastritis should be treated as for strong acids and alkalis (p. 96).

Reference

Temple AR, Veltri JC. Outcome of accidental ingestions of soaps, detergents and related household products. *Vet Hum Toxicol* 1979; **21** Suppl: 31–32.

CAMPHOR

General considerations

Camphor is extremely toxic and is present in a concentration of 20 per cent in camphorated oil and 10 per cent in camphor liniment, the respective solvents being cottonseed oil and alcohol. They are over-the-counter skin applications used to produce local warmth. Poisoning is usually the result of accidental ingestion, often in mistake for cod liver oil or castor oil. Camphor is lipid-soluble, rapidly absorbed and metabolised in the liver.

Features

Symptoms start within about an hour of ingestion and comprise burning in the epigastrium, nausea and vomiting. The patient may become excited with delirium and hallucinations. Signs of heightened neuromuscular excitability often precede convulsions which are common. Coma may supervene. Albuminuria and mild hyperbilirubinaemia without raised transaminases have been reported rarely.

Treatment

The stomach should be emptied as soon as possible. Agitation and convulsions should be treated with intravenous diazepam and supportive measures should be instituted to protect the airway and raise the blood pressure. Very severe poisoning has been treated by haemodialysis against soybean oil and by resin haemoperfusion but the value of these procedures is extremely doubtful.

Reference

Kopelman R, Miller S, Kelly R, Sunshine I. Camphor intoxication treated by resin hemoperfusion. *JAMA* 1979; **241**: 727–728.

CANNABIS

General considerations

Cannabis, the Indian hemp plant *(Cannabis sativa)*, contains several active constituents known as tetrahydrocannabinols. Cannabis resin (hashish) is obtained from the flowering top of the plant while the less potent leaves are termed marihuana, grass or pot. Cannabis is usually smoked or ingested but there have been occasional reports of intravenous injection of a 'tea' brewed from the plant. Very rarely intoxication may result from the rupture of ingested contraceptive sheaths in which the drug is being smuggled.

Features

The effects of cannabis are more readily controlled if it is smoked rather than ingested. Using the former route symptoms start within 10–20 minutes and last about 3 hours while with the latter the onset may be delayed up to 2 hours and persist for up to 6 hours. The symptoms are very variable. Initially there may be mild anxiety and excitement followed by a feeling of calmness, euphoria and uncontrollable laughter. Perception of colour and sound is often enhanced. Drowsiness and sleep follow. The only physical features may be an irritating, unproductive cough, dry mouth, tachycardia and conjunctival suffusion. On occasions, some individuals react with panic which may lead to hospital referral.

Intravenous injection of cannabis tea has much more serious consequences. Nausea, vomiting, abdominal pain and watery diarrhoea develop rapidly and are accompanied by rigors, fever, hypotension and shock. Renal impairment, cholestatic jaundice, muscle pain and weakness may become apparent over the next few days. The alterations in perception and cerebral function seen after cannabis has been smoked or ingested are strangely absent. A polymorph leukocytosis and thrombocytopenia may be found and hypoglycaemia has been reported. The ECG may show ischaemic changes.

Treatment

Treatment is usually unnecessary when cannabis has been inhaled or ingested. Panic reactions usually respond to reassurance and sedation with diazepam. Intravenous fluids and symptomatic measures are all that can be done for patients poisoned with intravenous cannabis.

References

Dassel PM, Punjabi E. Ingested marihuana-filled balloons. *Gastroenterology* 1979; **76**: 166–169.

Farber SJ, Huertas VE. Intravenously injected marihuana syndrome. *Arch Intern Med* 1976; **136**: 337–339.

Mims RB, Lee JH. Adverse effects of intravenous cannabis tea. *J Natl Med Assoc* 1977; **69**: 491–495.

Payne RJ, Brand SN. The toxicity of intravenously used marihuana. *JAMA* 1975; **233**: 351–354.

CARBAMAZEPINE

General considerations

Carbamazepine is used in the treatment of epilepsy and trigeminal neuralgia. Acute overdosage has been reported infrequently.

Features

Drowsiness, ataxia and incoordination are followed by loss of consciousness. A divergent strabismus may be present during coma and disappear with recovery. Muscle tone is often increased and opisthotonos and convulsions may occur. When roused, patients tend to react violently and thrash around in bed. Respiration is rarely depressed. Many of the adverse reactions to therapeutic doses of carbamazepine have not been reported after acute overdosage.

Treatment

There is no specific treatment for carbamazepine poisoning. Most patients should recover with supportive measures alone but the rate of recovery may be slow because of the long plasma half-life of the drug.

References

Drenck NE, Risbo A. Carbamazepine poisoning, a surprisingly severe case. *Anaesth Intens Care* 1980; **8**: 203–205.

Zeeuw RA, Westenberg HGM, Vander Kleijn E, Gimbrere JSF. An unusual case of carbamazepine poisoning with near fatal relapse after two days. *Vet Hum Toxicol* 1979; **21** Suppl: 95–97.

CARBON MONOXIDE

General considerations

Carbon monoxide was formerly one of the most important causes of accidental and suicidal poisoning deaths because of its presence in coal gas and car exhaust fumes. Though the latter is still occasionally a problem in clinical practice, the nationwide conversion to natural gas for domestic purposes has very considerably reduced the number of deaths from carbon monoxide poisoning. However, serious poisoning still occurs though the causes are now more subtle. Many cases arise from the incomplete combustion of methane, butane and propane either because they have been used in a confined atmosphere (e.g. caravans) where ventilation may have been deliberately reduced to increase warmth or because the appliance is faulty or vents are blocked. The use of charcoal grills and paint removers containing methylene chloride in confined spaces has also caused carbon monoxide poisoning. The latter may be particularly serious since the metabolism of methylene chloride to carbon monoxide continues after exposure has ceased.

Carbon monoxide is bound to haemoglobin to form carboxyhaemoglobin, the affinity of haemoglobin for carbon monoxide being 200–300 times greater than for oxygen. It also combines with cytochrome oxidases. As a result it is generally accepted that the toxicity of carbon monoxide is mainly due to hypoxia. The latter explains the high morbidity and mortality of carbon monoxide in elderly patients, many of whom have pre-existing atherosclerosis.

Features

The early features of carbon monoxide poisoning are headache, dizziness, nausea and vomiting. The vomitus may contain altered blood. Coma supervenes and is accompanied by hyperventilation, hypotension, increased muscle tone, hyperreflexia, clonus, extensor plantar responses, piloerection and shivering. Contrary to popular belief the skin seldom shows the cherry-pink colour of carboxyhaemoglobin during life; a combination of central and peripheral cyanosis is much more likely. Skin blistering and muscle necrosis may occur if the patient has been lying for some time, but renal failure (secondary to myoglobinuria) and myositis ossificans are very rare. Retinal haemorrhages and papilloedema secondary to hypoxic cerebral oedema may be present.

Arterial blood gas analysis usually shows a metabolic acidosis with a normal oxygen tension but reduced oxygen saturation and there may be electrocardiographic evidence of myocardial ischaemia.

Treatment

The first steps are to remove the patient from the toxic atmosphere and ensure that the airway, ventilation and blood pressure are adequate. The oxygen concentration of the inspired air should be increased as far as possible but there is no need to refer for hyperbaric oxygen therapy unless carboxyhaemoglobin concentrations are very high and the facility is readily available. Any metabolic acidosis will usually respond to correction of hypoxia but, if severe, intravenous bicarbonate may be given. Care should be taken not to give too much fluid intravenously, particularly in the elderly and in those whose ECGs show ischaemic changes. Mannitol and dexamethasone should be given if cerebral oedema is present (p. 51). Assisted ventilation may occasionally be necessary in severe poisoning.

Prognosis

Patients who reach hospital alive are likely to survive though some, particularly the elderly, may die from myocardial infarction and CNS damage. Parietal lobe lesions, parkinsonism and akinetic mutism have been reported in survivors. Others appear to recover rapidly but after a few days develop permanent neuro-psychiatric symptoms including inability to concentrate, recent memory impairment, intellectual deterioration and personality change as manifested by irritability, moodiness and a tendency to be aggressive and impulsive. The presence of low density areas in the globus pallidus shown by computerised tomography of the brain on admission to hospital has been shown to correlate with a poor outcome.

References

Hopkinson JM, Pearce PJ, Oliver JS. Carbon monoxide poisoning mimicking gastroenteritis. *Br Med J* 1980; **281**: 214–215.

Jackson DL, Menges H. Accidental carbon monoxide poisoning. *JAMA* 1980; **243**: 772–774.

Myers RAM, Linberg SE, Cowley RA. Carbon monoxide poisoning: the injury and its treatment. *JACEP* 1979; **8**: 479–484.

Sawada Y, Takahashi M, Ohashi N, et al. Computerised tomography as an indication of long-term outcome after acute carbon monoxide poisoning. *Lancet* 1980; **1**: 783–784.

CARBON TETRACHLORIDE AND RELATED CHLORINATED HYDROCARBONS

Carbon tetrachloride	Tetrachloroethylene
Tetrachloroethane	Trichloroethylene

General considerations

These compounds are used extensively in industry as solvents and dry-cleaning and degreasing agents. Carbon tetrachloride was formerly used in fire extinguishers and trichloroethylene as an anaesthetic. Severe poisoning is uncommon; it may result from inhalation during use in confined spaces or after accidental or intentional ingestion.

Features

All of these hydrocarbons produce major CNS effects with excitement in the early stages followed by drowsiness, ataxia and coma. If the concentration in the atmosphere is very high death may occur and pulmonary oedema is frequently found at autopsy.

The other major toxic effects are on the liver and kidneys. Carbon tetrachloride, however, is considerably more toxic than the others and there is doubt as to whether trichloroethylene causes any degree of liver damage. Carbon tetrachloride is metabolised by hepatic microsomal oxidase systems and toxicity is due to a highly reactive intermediate metabolite. Enzyme induction increases the rate of production of the metabolite and probably explains the long-recognised particular susceptibility of chronic alcoholics to carbon tetrachloride hepatotoxicity. The pathogenesis and clinical course of the centrilobular necrosis is similar to that of acute paracetamol overdose (p. 157).

Renal tubular necrosis may also occur.

Treatment

When poisoning has been the result of inhalation the patient should be removed from the toxic environment. If the solvent has been ingested the stomach should be emptied. In either case supportive measures should be instituted if consciousness is impaired and liver function, urine production and the plasma urea and creatinine should be monitored daily for 4 days.

There is no readily available method of assessing the severity of poisoning or predicting liver damage though possibly the degree of CNS depression might be the best guide. If carbon tetrachloride poisoning is considered severe and the patient can be treated within ten hours N-acetylcysteine should be given as for paracetamol overdosage (p. 162) to prevent liver damage. This treatment is also appropriate for poisoning with the other chlorinated hydrocarbons, which cause liver necrosis. Renal failure should be managed conventionally.

CHLORAL HYDRATE AND RELATED HYPNOTICS

Chloral hydrate	Dichloralphenazone
Chloral betaine	Triclofos

General considerations

Chloral hydrate is one of the oldest hypnotics. The other drugs listed above are rapidly broken down in the stomach to yield chloral hydrate and therefore have identical effects. Chloral hydrate is very rapidly metabolised by alcohol dehydrogenase to trichloroethanol which is then oxidised to trichloracetic acid. Poisoning with these compounds is uncommon. Chronic use may lead to physical and psychological dependence.

Features

Chloral hydrate irritates the oesophageal and gastric mucosae causing heartburn, nausea and vomiting. In other respects however, most of the features of overdosage are similar to those of ethanol poisoning with coma, hypotension, vasodilatation and respiratory depression. The most serious complications are supraventricular and ventricular dysrhythmias leading to cardiac arrest. It has been estimated that ectopic beats should be expected in 25 per cent of cases. Rarely, albuminuria and jaundice may occur.

Treatment

The stomach should be emptied if fifteen tablets or more have been ingested within the preceding 4 hours. The great majority of cases will require no more than supportive care. The cardiac rhythm should be monitored but though dysrhythmias complicating chloral hydrate poisoning appear alarming they often terminate spontaneously. If they cause haemodynamic problems, however, they respond dramatically to practolol.

Haemodialysis has been shown to considerably shorten the plasma half-life of trichloroethanol (it should be noted that chloral hydrate is so rapidly metabolised that it is not present in significant quantities in plasma) and may be helpful in rare patients who are very severely poisoned. Haemoperfusion may be even more effective.

References

Gustafson A, Svensson SE, Ugander L. Cardiac arrhythmias in chloral hydrate poisoning. *Acta Med Scand* 1977; **201**: 227–230.
Stalker NE, Gambertoglio JG, Fukumitsu CJ, Naughton JL, Benet LZ. Acute massive chloral hydrate intoxication treated with hemodialysis: a clinical pharmacokinetic analysis. *J Clin Pharmacol* 1978; **18**: 136–142.
Wiseman HM, Hampel G. Cardiac arrhythmias due to chloral hydrate poisoning. *Br Med J* 1978; **2**: 960.

CHLORATES

General considerations

Poisoning with chlorates is uncommon and is usually due to ingestion of sodium chlorate which is available as a weedkiller. Chlorates are powerful oxidising agents.

Features

Chlorates irritate the gastrointestinal tract causing nausea, vomiting, diarrhoea and abdominal pain. Haematological effects, including intravascular haemolysis and methaemoglobinaemia are common. As a result the blood may be chocolate coloured and the plasma and urine dark. The patient will be cyanosed. Jaundice and oliguric renal failure may develop. A leukocytosis is common. Death may occur in the acute phase due to hypoxia secondary to severe methaemoglobinaemia or from hyperkalaemia.

Treatment

The stomach should be emptied if the patient presents within 4 hours of ingestion of the chlorate. Methaemoglobinaemia can be corrected by slow intravenous injection of methylene blue (0.1 ml of a 1% solution/kg body weight) which may have to be repeated. Absorbic acid is of no value. Blood transfusion may be necessary if there has been severe haemolysis but will be of limited value if chlorate is still present in the circulation. Haemodialysis will remove chlorate in severe poisoning and may be necessary for the management of renal failure.

Reference

Helliwell M, Nunn J. Mortality in sodium chlorate poisoning. *Br Med J* 1979; **1**: 1119.

CHLORINE

General considerations

Chlorine is widely used in industrial processes including water purification and the manufacture of hydrochloric acid, bleaches and plastics. Domestic exposure may occur if household bleaches are mixed with acidic lavatory cleaners or during school chemistry experiments. In addition to hydrochloric and hypochlorous acids, the reaction of chlorine with water produces several toxic unstable oxidising agents. Inhalation of chlorine results in patchy necrosis of the respiratory mucosa at all levels and acute pulmonary oedema.

Features

Symptoms usually start within a few hours, the speed of onset being dependent on the magnitude of exposure. Lacrimation, conjunctivitis and cough are early symptoms and are followed by breathlessness, wheeze and expectoration of white frothy sputum which may become blood-stained. There may be hoarseness due to laryngeal oedema. Clinical examination usually reveals tachypnoea, and central cyanosis with crepitations and rhonchi throughout the lungs. Patchy and confluent areas of pulmonary oedema are present radiologically. Arterial blood gas analysis usually shows some degree of hypoxia and perhaps a metabolic acidosis but hypercapnia does not occur except at an advanced stage. A polymorph leukocytosis is common. Death is due to gross hypoxia and coma.

Treatment

The first step is to remove the patient from the toxic atmosphere. All but those who have been minimally exposed should be observed for 12 hours or advised to report immediately should they develop respiratory symptoms. Oxygen therapy will be necessary if hypoxia is present. Bronchodilators may relieve bronchospasm but, since the pulmonary oedema is non-cardiac in aetiology, digoxin and diuretics are ineffective. Prednisolone 60 mg daily (or equivalent) should be given until symptoms have disappeared and there has been radiological clearing, then withdrawn over about two weeks. In severe cases, endotracheal intubation and assisted ventilation may be necessary if hypoxia cannot be adequately corrected by oxygen by face mask or if hypercapnia occurs.

Reference

Hedges JR, Morrissey WL. Acute chlorine gas exposure. *JACEP* 1979; **8**: 59–63.

CHLORMETHIAZOLE

General considerations

Chlormethiazole is a potent CNS depressant which is chemically related to vitamin B_1 and is used as a hypnotic and for the prevention and treatment of the alcohol withdrawal syndrome. Unfortunately it is frequently prescribed long-term to alcoholics who are continuing to drink. The practice is pointless and potentially dangerous since alcohol potentiates the CNS depressant effects of the drug and dependence on chlormethiazole commonly occurs. Chlormethiazole is extensively metabolised in the liver to inactive compounds, metabolism being impaired in the elderly and those with advanced cirrhosis.

Features

The features of chlormethiazole overdosage are similar to those of barbiturate poisoning with impairment of consciousness leading to deep coma, hypotension, hypothermia and respiratory depression in severe cases. There is hypotonia, hyporeflexia and normal or absent plantar responses. The pupils do not show any specific changes. Increased salivation has been noted in a significant number of cases and may predispose to aspiration pneumonia.

Treatment

The stomach should be emptied if more than fifteen dosage units have been ingested within the preceding 4 hours. Atropine may be given to counteract troublesome hypersalivation but is best avoided. Frequent pharyngeal suction and supportive care is all that is required for most cases. Forced diuresis would not be expected to be beneficial and the efficacy of haemodialysis and haemoperfusion has not been assessed. The latter may be the treatment of choice if the patient is severely poisoned and recovery of consciousness is a matter of great urgency.

Plasma chlormethiazole concentrations

The limited data available suggest that plasma chlormethiazole concentrations correlate poorly with clinical assessment of the severity of poisoning and they are therefore of limited value in routine management. Patients with plasma concentrations up to 36 mg/l (about 20 times those after a single therapeutic dose) have recovered uneventfully. Coma is usual with concentrations above 7 mg/l. It should be noted that assays performed by ultraviolet spectrophotometry may be non-specific and give spuriously high plasma concentrations.

Reference

Illingworth RN, Stewart MJ, Jarvie DR. Severe poisoning with chlormethiazole. *Br Med J* 1979; **2**: 902–903.

CHLOROQUINE

General considerations

Chloroquine is a derivative of 4-aminoquinoline and is used for the prophylaxis and treatment of malaria and in connective tissue disorders such as rheumatoid arthritis and systemic lupus erythematosus. The considerable toxicity of this drug in overdosage is not widely appreciated.

Features

Chloroquine is rapidly and almost completely absorbed after ingestion and symptoms may start within an hour. Nausea, vomiting and drowsiness occur early and may be followed by slurring of speech, agitation, breathlessness due to pulmonary oedema, convulsions and coma. The most serious toxic effects are on the heart where the quinidine-like action causes bradycardia, hypotension, QRS widening, ventricular ectopic beats, ventricular tachycardia and fibrillation. The interval between ingestion and cardiac arrest may be as short as 3 hours or even considerably less. In one series 50 per cent of patients who ingested 2.25 g or more of chloroquine base developed serious cardiac complications.

Treatment

The stomach should be emptied if the tablets have been ingested in the preceding 4 hours. Hypoxia, acid–base disturbances and hyperkalaemia should be sought and treated if necessary. Cardiac dysrhythmias should not be treated unless they are life-threatening since the administration of cardiac depressant anti-arrhythmic drugs to counteract the toxicity of another is illogical.

Tissue chloroquine concentrations are considerably higher than those in plasma and 70 per cent of the drug is slowly excreted unchanged in the urine. It has been suggested, but not proved, that forced acid diuresis will increase elimination. Possible benefit from this treatment is extremely unlikely and must be weighed against the risk of pulmonary oedema in a patient with impaired myocardial contractility.

Prognosis

Many patients severely poisoned with chloroquine are likely to have a cardiac arrest before reaching medical care. The absence of cardiac effects 4–6 hours after ingestion makes survival likely.

Reference

Britton WJ, Kevau IH. Intentional chloroquine overdosage. *Med J Aust* 1978; **2**: 407–410.

CHLORPROPAMIDE

General considerations

The oral hypoglycaemic agent, chlorpropamide, acts by stimulating insulin release from the pancreas and hyperinsulinaemia has been reported after overdosage. Chlorpropamide is said to be rapidly absorbed but after overdosage peak plasma concentrations may not be attained for up to 39 hours. About 90 per cent of chlorpropamide is protein bound and approximately 80 per cent is metabolised in the liver, the plasma half-life being 35–40 hours after therapeutic doses and probably much longer after overdosage.

Features

The features of chlorpropamide overdosage are those of profound hypoglycaemia with impairment of consciousness, hypertonia, hyperreflexia, clonus and extensor plantar responses. The pupils may or may not be dilated and convulsions may occur. Paradoxically the skin is usually dry. Because the plasma half-life of the drug is so long hypoglycaemia may be protracted or recur despite carbohydrate intake at any time up to five days after self-poisoning. Cerebral oedema, neurogenic diabetes insipidus and death has occurred.

Treatment

Urgent steps should be taken to correct hypoglycaemia before proceeding to gastric lavage. However, even very large amounts of intravenous dextrose may not be sufficient to restore normal blood glucose concentrations or abolish the features of poisoning. Glucagon has been recommended if the patient presents within a few hours of ingestion but is unlikely to be effective after 24–36 hours because hepatic glycogen stores may have been depleted. Both glucose and glucagon will further stimulate insulin release and exacerbate the tendency to hypoglycaemia. Diazoxide is a more rational therapy as it blocks insulin release and raises plasma catecholamine concentrations. Intravenous therapy may be required initially (1.25 mg/kg given over one hour) and repeated six-hourly. Such doses do not cause hypotension. The plasma potassium will tend to fall and must be monitored carefully. Elimination of the poison cannot be enhanced by forced diuresis or haemodialysis. Convulsions should respond to correction of the blood glucose but if this is not immediately possible, diazepam may be necessary. Cerebral oedema should be treated conventionally. Once the acute phase is over, diazoxide may be given orally (5 mg/kg body weight in two or three divided doses daily) until there is no risk of hypoglycaemia.

References

Jacobs RF, Nix RA, Paulus TE, Kiel EA, Fiser RH. Intravenous infusion of diazoxide in the treatment of chlorpropamide-induced hypoglycaemia. *J Pediatr* 1978; **93**: 801–803.

Pfeifer MA, Wolter CF, Samols E. Management of chlorpropamide induced hypoglycaemia with diazoxide. *South Med J* 1978; **71**: 606–608.

CIMETIDINE

General considerations

This drug is a histamine H_2 receptor antagonist and is being increasingly used for the treatment of duodenal ulceration. Inevitably, increasing numbers of self-poisonings with cimetidine can be expected.

Features

Cimetidine appears to be remarkably non-toxic in acute overdosage. Patients with plasma concentrations of cimetidine up to 57 mg/l (60 times the peak values obtained after one therapeutic dose) have been reported to have no symptoms other than drowsiness and dryness of the mouth.

Treatment

Treatment is unnecessary. A good urinary output should be ensured since cimetidine is excreted largely unchanged in the urine.

Reference

Illingworth RN, Jarvie DR. Absence of toxicity in cimetidine overdosage. *Br Med J* 1979; **1**: 453–454.

CLONIDINE

General considerations

Clonidine stimulates peripheral alpha-adrenergic receptors and also has central nervous system actions. Low-dose formulations are used for the treatment of migraine and menopausal flushing while higher-dose formulations are used for the management of hypertension. Poisoning is more common in children than adults and usually involves the low-dose preparation, probably because of its greater availability, attractive blue colour and sugar coating.

Features

Drowsiness and impairment of consciousness are the commonest findings. The pupils may be constricted and unresponsive to light. Bradycardia is also common and hypotension is present in about 20 per cent of cases. Much less frequently, severe hypertension occurs when peripheral effects predominate. Other features include pallor, respiratory depression, cardiac dysrhythmias and convulsions.

Treatment

There is no specific treatment for clonidine overdosage. Supportive measures are generally all that are required. The bradycardia usually responds to atropine. Alpha-adrenergic blocking drugs such as phentolamine and tolazoline have been shown experimentally to reverse the central and peripheral actions of clonidine but their value in human intoxication is unknown. They may, however, have a role in the management of severe poisoning, especially in the treatment of serious hypertension.

More than half the absorbed dose of clonidine is excreted unchanged in the urine in 24 hours but the value of forced diuresis and other measures intended to enhance elimination has not been critically assessed. They will seldom be indicated.

Prognosis

Considerable clinical improvement can be expected within 12 hours of ingestion and in most cases recovery will be complete within 48 hours.

References

Grabert B, Conner CS, Rumack BH, Peterson RG. Clonidine-recurrent apnea following overdose. *Drug Intelligence and Clin Pharm* 1980; **13**: 778–780.

Stein B, Volans GN. Dixarit overdose: the problem of attractive tablets. *Br Med J* 1978; **2**: 667–668.

COLCHICINE

General considerations

Colchicine poisoning is uncommon and is usually the result of deliberate self-poisoning with colchicine tablets or ingestion of parts of the meadow saffron, *Colchicum autumnale,* though serious poisoning due to therapeutic misadventure has occurred. The mortality is high, particularly when the ingested dose exceeds 40 mg. Colchicine is a direct cell poison which preferentially damages cells that divide most rapidly.

Features

Symptoms usually start after 3–4 hours with vomiting, nausea, abdominal pain and diarrhoea, the latter being so profuse that the bowel motion resembles the rice-water stool of cholera. Bowel activity is reduced. Dehydration, oliguria, hypotension and shock follow rapidly. There may be burning in the throat with ulceration of the buccal mucosa. Muscle pain, tenderness and weakness, confusion, breathlessness (due to pulmonary oedema) and ventilatory failure often develop after 2-3 days.

Numerous laboratory abnormalities occur during severe colchicine poisoning. In some cases there is an initial polymorph leukocytosis but after as little as a few hours or as long as 4 days profound neutropenia and thrombocytopenia usually develop. As a result severely poisoned patients usually die from infection and haemorrhagic complications. Mild hepatocellular damage and renal failure are common. The serum amylase may be elevated though it is uncertain whether it is derived from pancreas or gut. Persistent hypokalaemia may be a problem and arterial blood gas analysis frequently shows a metabolic acidosis with hypoxia.

Paralytic ileus and convulsions have been described relatively late in the course of colchicine poisoning and alopecia does not usually become apparent till about 10 days after ingestion. By about the sixth day after poisoning the white cell and platelet counts begin to rise and may overshoot normal levels. Peripheral neuropathy is common in survivors.

Treatment

The uninformed physician may be lulled into an unjustified sense of security by the delay in onset of symptoms in colchicine poisoning. However, patients clearly require constant and prolonged supervision. The serious toxicity of colchicine justifies gastric lavage regardless of the number of tablets taken. Adequate intravenous fluids and electrolytes are essential at an early stage to replace gastrointestinal losses and maintain the blood pressure and urinary output. Unfortunately there is no method of enhancing the elimination of colchicine. Complications must be sought and treated as they arise. Antibiotics and platelet transfusions may be necessary.

Reference

Jarvie D, Park J, Stewart MJ. Estimation of colchicine in a poisoned patient by using high performance liquid chromatography. *Clin Toxicol* 1979; **14**: 375–381.

CONTRACEPTIVE PREPARATIONS

General considerations

There are many different oral contraceptive preparations but most comprise a progestogen in combination with a synthetic oestrogen. They are virtually non-toxic.

Features

The majority of patients will have no symptoms. Nausea and vomiting may occur but settle rapidly. Vaginal withdrawal bleeding may occur in pre-pubertal girls.

Treatment

Usually no treatment is required.

CORROSIVES

Strong acids	*Strong alkalis*
Hydrochloric acid	Ammonia
Nitric acid	Lye
Sulphuric acid	Potassium hydroxide
	Sodium hydroxide

General considerations

Many poisons other than the strong acids and alkalis listed above have corrosive effects on the gastrointestinal tract but their other actions justify considering them separately. They include iron salts, paraquat, phenol, oxalic acid and mercuric chloride.

Poisoning with strong acids and alkalis is uncommon in the United Kingdom but not infrequent in the United States where they are available for domestic use as drain and oven cleaners (particularly lye, a non-specific term for a mixture of sodium and potassium hydroxides). In consequence, accidental poisoning with corrosives is most frequent in children, though accidental and deliberate self-poisoning in adults is not uncommon. Dilute sulphuric acid is also available as battery acid. Clinitest tablets, which contain sodium hydroxide, are occasionally ingested by diabetics who have misunderstood or not been told clearly by their doctors what to do with them.

Features

The ingestion of strong acids and alkalis produces almost immediate burning pain in the lips, mouth, throat, substernal region and epigastrium. Vomiting occurs very rapidly and may recur repeatedly with the vomitus becoming blood-stained. Hypersalivation is common. Shock and melaena may develop in severe poisoning. The patient may look pale and burns may be visible on the hands and face. A few patients escape buccal burns but most show red, oedematous areas with superficial desquamation. Only a small minority show deep destruction of buccal tissues.

The development of oesophageal or gastric necrosis depends to some extent on whether an acid or alkali has been ingested. Alkalis commonly produce oesophageal burns but only about 20 per cent of patients have gastric lesions. In contrast, the oesophageal mucosa is relatively resistant to acids whereas the gastric mucosa, particularly in the region of the antrum, is especially vulnerable.

Following alkali ingestion about a third of patients with mouth burns have similar lesions in the oesophagus. Oesophageal necrosis may be present in about 15 per cent of those without buccal abnormalities. In severe cases the oesophagus may be perforated leading to mediastinitis but this is more likely to be a complication of oesophagoscopy. The major long-term complication is oesophageal stricture formation.

Gastric damage due to acids can be equally severe with coagulative necrosis of the mucosa, principally in the antrum, with haemorrhage and gangrene (which may involve the whole stomach) and peritonitis. Antral strictures usually become apparent 3 weeks to 3 months after ingestion or even much later.

Treatment

Every case should be referred to hospital for assessment. Milk should be given as a first aid measure to help neutralise the corrosive but in severe cases the patient is unlikely to be able to retain it. There is no merit in wasting time searching for citric acid, vinegar or sodium bicarbonate. Gastric lavage is contraindicated. Analgesics and intravenous fluids or blood are often required and metabolic acidosis should be sought and treated appropriately.

Oesophagoscopy in the acute phase is hazardous and best avoided though it has been advocated by some workers to exclude the presence of oesophageal burns so that hospitalisation is no longer than necessary. If it is considered essential, it should only be performed by an experienced endoscopist and the instrument should not be passed beyond the first burn since attempts to progress further are associated with a greatly increased incidence of perforation. Contrast X-rays of the oesophagus are less helpful in identifying burns. Patients with mediastinitis should, if possible, be managed conservatively. However, surgery, including resection, may be necessary if there is perforation or serious haemorrhage from the stomach. It is preferable to avoid surgery in the acute phase if at all possible.

Not surprisingly, the alleged benefits of corticosteroids in the prevention of stricture formation have not been confirmed by controlled trials but it is generally held that they are useful if given as early as possible, in high doses, being tailed off over about 3 weeks.

References

Adams JT, Skucas J. Corrosive jejunitis due to ingestion of nitric acid. *Am J Surg* 1980; **139**:282–285.

Cello JP, Fogel RP, Boland R. Liquid caustic ingestion. *Arch Intern Med* 1980; **140**:501–504.

Cochran ST, Fonkalsrud EW, Gyepes MT. Complete obstruction of the gastric antrum in children following acid ingestion. *Arch Surg* 1978; **113**:308–310.

Mallory A, Schaefer JW. Clinitest ingestion. *Br Med J* 1977; **2**:105–107.

Marshall F. Caustic burns of the esophagus: ten year results of aggressive care. *South Med J* 1979; **72**:1236–1237.

COTONEASTER

General considerations

Several varieties of this garden shrub and the related species, pyracantha, are cultivated in Europe and North America. During the autumn the plants carry numerous attractive scarlet berries which have a fleshy exterior and a central stone which contains the seeds. The seeds contain cyanogenic glycosides but it is highly improbable that a sufficient number would be eaten to cause serious symptoms.

Features

Most children will have no symptoms. Others may vomit or develop abdominal pain or diarrhoea.

Treatment

Treatment is usually superfluous. If a large number of berries has been ingested the stomach should be emptied. Symptomatic measures may rarely be required.

CYANIDE

General considerations

Cyanides are widely used in industry but with such stringent precautions that poisoning is extremely uncommon. However, sodium cyanide is used in less well controlled circumstances for the elimination of colonies of rabbits. Hydrogen cyanide is produced in fires involving the decomposition of polyurethane foams and from the hydrolysis of laetrile (amygdalin), a cyanogenic glycoside contained in the kernels of apricots, cherries and other plants of the *Rosacea* family.

The cyanide ion binds strongly to the ferric component of cytochrome oxidase, effectively preventing utilisation of oxygen by cells and causing hypoxia. Anaerobic glycolysis and severe metabolic acidosis result.

Features

Most of the clinical features of cyanide poisoning are due to severe hypoxia although cyanosis is not present. The odour of bitter almonds on the breath is said to be characteristic but it is not always present and even if it were, it is questionable how many doctors would recognise it. Early symptoms of poisoning include feelings of anxiety, headache, dizziness, palpitations, weakness and drowsiness. Consciousness will be lost in severe cases and convulsions and cerebral oedema may be problems. Cardio-respiratory abnormalities may become prominent with breathlessness, tachypnoea, hypotension, pulmonary oedema, bradycardia, conduction defects and dysrhythmias. Arterial blood gas analysis shows a metabolic acidosis.

Treatment

When hydrogen cyanide has been inhaled the patient must be removed from the contaminated atmosphere. The importance of supportive measures to establish and maintain adequate airway and ventilation cannot be emphasised too strongly. Oxygen in high concentrations must be given and metabolic acidosis should be sought and corrected. These measures may be sufficient to improve the blood pressure but the use of vasopressor agents is contraindicated because of their ability to cause dysrhythmias in the presence of hypoxia. When cyanide has been ingested, gastric aspiration and lavage should be carried out. The use of a 5% solution of sodium thiosulphate for lavage has been recommended but the procedure should not be delayed if this is not immediately available. Likewise 200 ml of 25% sodium thiosulphate may be left in the stomach at the end of lavage.

Contrary to popular belief, most patients do not die within minutes of cyanide poisoning. Indeed many survive severe poisoning for hours before being given antidotes and others have recovered uneventfully with no more than the supportive therapy described above. These facts in no way belittle the importance of antidotes but merely emphasise that their role is complementary. Because the antidotes are potentially dangerous in the absence of cyanide ions the diagnosis must be beyond doubt before they are given and clinically the poisoning should be moderate or severe (i.e. with impairment of consciousness). The antidote of choice is dicobalt edetate (Kelocyanor) 600 mg intravenously. A further 300 mg may be given a few minutes later if the first dose does not produce a satisfactory response. The recommendation that it should be followed by 25 g of glucose intravenously is harmless but valueless.

If dicobalt edetate is not available the older intravenous regime of sodium nitrite (10 ml of a 3% solution given over 3 min) followed by sodium thiosulphate (50 ml of a 25% solution given over 10 min) should be used. For children the dose of nitrite should be 10 mg/kg immediately and 5 mg/kg after 30 min if necessary. Methaemoglobin produced by sodium nitrite binds cyanide ions avidly to form cyanmethaemoglobin and facilitates the transfer of cyanide bound to tissue cytochrome oxidases to haemoglobin where it is less harmful. Thiosulphate provides the sulphur to combine with cyanide via rhodanese to form non-toxic thiocyanate which is then excreted in the urine. The rationale of the first aid measure involving the inhalation of amyl nitrite is similar but it is doubtful if sufficient methaemoglobin could be produced in this way without causing serious hypotension and it is not recommended.

References

Braico KT, Humbert JR, Terplan KL, Lehotay JM. Laetrile intoxication. *New Engl J Med* 1979; **300**:238–240.
Bryson DD. Cyanide poisoning. *Br Med J* 1978; **1**:92.
Graham DL, Laman D, Theodore J, et al. Acute cyanide poisoning complicated by lactic acidosis and pulmonary edema. *Arch Intern Med* 1977; **137**:1051–1055.

DIEFFENBACHIA, MONSTERA AND PHILODENDRON

General considerations

Dieffenbachia, Monstera and *Philodendron* are members of the *Araceae* family of plants (frequently referred to as aroids) and are commonly grown throughout Europe and North America as ornamental house plants. They share a common mode of toxicity though only the genus *Dieffenbachia* has been studied extensively. All parts of the plant contain specialised cells in which there are bundles (raphides) of needle-like crystals of calcium oxalate. When the plant is chewed the sharp crystals disrupt the mucus membrane allowing a proteolytic enzyme to penetrate. The latter is thought to be responsible for most of the ensuing inflammation.

Poisoning with these plants is most common in children.

Features

Chewing the leaves or stems of the plants almost immediately causes intense burning pain in the lips and mouth and hypersalivation. The buccal mucosa, lips, tongue and palate become inflamed and swollen due to oedema making speech difficult or impossible. The latter has earned *Dieffenbachia* the popular name 'dumb cane'. In severe cases acute laryngeal oedema may develop and cause serious respiratory obstruction, especially in small children. Retrosternal pain and oesophageal necrosis has been reported in an adult.

The oedema usually subsides within 3 or 4 days but pain may persist longer.

Treatment

Treatment is symptomatic. Some relief may be obtained from sucking ice and milk or antacids have been recommended. Serious respiratory obstruction due to laryngeal oedema may require endotracheal intubation (if possible) or tracheostomy. Corticosteroids may be given but their value in settling the oedema has not been assessed.

DIGOXIN AND DIGITOXIN

General considerations

While therapeutic intoxication with cardiac glycosides is common, acute massive overdosage is relatively rare, presumably reflecting the very small number of people needing these drugs in the age groups in which self-poisoning is most common. However acute digoxin and digitoxin poisoning occasionally occurs in children and adults whose hearts are normal.

Digoxin poisoning has been reported from Britain, Scandinavia and North America while most accounts of digitoxin poisoning have come from the European continent.

Overdosage is usually the result of ingestion but self-poisoning by the intravenous route has been described.

Features

Nausea, vomiting, diarrhoea and extreme wretchedness are early features and drowsiness, confusion and delirium are not uncommon. Pale, cold extremities and hypotension indicate reduced cardiac output.

The most important toxic effects of the cardiac glycosides are on the heart. It is generally accepted that membrane ATPase is inhibited with resultant increase in intracellular sodium concentrations and leakage of potassium from the cells. Hyperkalaemia is common in severe cases. In the early stages of poisoning the loss of intracellular potassium reduces the resting membrane potential and increases the excitability of the myocardium. However, if the membrane potential is further reduced by continuing potassium leakage, excitability is impaired since the rapid inflow phase of the action potential is diminished in proportion to the resting membrane potential.

Sinus arrest and sino-atrial block are occasionally encountered but the commonest problem is sinus bradycardia with PR prolongation progressing to varying degrees of A-V block and A-V dissociation. As a consequence junctional escape rhythms may develop. His bundle electrography has shown that the block occurs in the A-V node but there is dispute about slowing of conduction in the bundle of His and the Purkinje system. Though ventricular ectopics, bigeminy, ventricular tachycardia and paroxysmal atrial tachycardia may occur the evidence suggests that they are more frequent with therapeutic intoxication than in acute overdosage in patients with normal hearts.

In addition to hyperkalaemia there may be hypoxia and a metabolic acidosis due to impaired tissue perfusion.

Treatment

The stomach should be emptied if more than ten tablets have been ingested within 4 hours. While oral activated charcoal is of doubtful value in most poisonings, it has no adverse effects and its use in potentially serious poisoning with cardiac glycosides does not require justification. It should be given regularly (vomiting permitting) until signs of serious toxicity have passed, to interrupt entero-hepatic circulation of the drug. The latter is more important with digitoxin than digoxin. Cholestyramine (4 g orally four times daily) or colestipol, a steroid-binding resin (5 g orally four times daily) may be used as alternatives to activated charcoal.

The plasma potassium and urea should be measured urgently and hyperkalaemia (>6.0 mmol/l) treated initially by giving glucose (25 g intravenously) and soluble insulin (10 units intravenously). Arterial blood gas analysis is advised if there is any suspicion of impaired tissue perfusion and hypoxia and metabolic acidosis corrected appropriately.

The cardiac rhythm must be monitored continuously. Sinus bradycardia, ventricular ectopics, A-V block and sino-atrial stand-still or block are often reduced or abolished by atropine (1.2 mg intravenously as required). Ventricular ectopics alone should not be treated unless cardiac output is impaired. Ventricular tachydys-rhythmias are best treated with lignocaine or practolol. Verapamil has theoretical advantages over practolol in the management of supraventricular tachycardia but its value in acute digoxin overdos-age has not been adequately tested. Direct current countershock should be avoided if at all possible. Failure to achieve a satisfactory cardiac output by drug therapy in patients with bradycardia, A-V block or sinus arrest is an indication for insertion of a right ventricular pacing catheter. It has also been suggested that this should be done prophylactically if severe hyperkalaemia is present since this may presage the onset of serious bradydysrhythmias. The pacing threshold tends to rise with increasing severity of poisoning and in the worst cases pacing may fail to initiate contraction.

Though a variety of techniques have been tried in attempts to enhance the elimination of cardiac glycosides they have met with little success because most of the drug is tissue-bound and plasma concentrations are low. Digoxin is excreted through the kidneys but forced diuresis does not increase its clearance except in the first 4–6 hours after a large overdose before distribution of the drug has been completed. Even in these optimal circumstances, however, only very small quantities of drug can be recovered. Exchange transfusion, peritoneal dialysis and haemodialysis are of no value and though claims have been made for the usefulness of charcoal and resin haemoperfusion adequate confirmatory data is lacking. It would be surprising if they could quickly remove toxicologically significant quantities of a drug which has such a large volume of distribution.

The most promising therapeutic approach to severe digoxin intoxication involves giving purified Fab fragments of digoxin antibodies. Their use in one case produced rapid return of sinus rhythm and correction of hyperkalaemia and decline in plasma concentrations of free digoxin over a few hours. Unfortunately digoxin antibodies are not widely available and are very expensive. The poisons information service should be contacted for advice.

Prognosis

Acute digoxin overdosage carries a mortality of 10–20 per cent. Factors indicating a poor prognosis include hyperkalaemia, failure to respond to drug therapy and a rising threshold for myocardial pacing. Recovery takes several days because of the long plasma half-life of cardiac glycosides (about 36 hours for digoxin and seven days for digitoxin).

Plasma digoxin concentrations

Though plasma digoxin concentrations of up to 52 µg/l have been found after acute overdosage, measurement in the acute phase is of no value in management.

References

Bismuth C, Motte G, Conso F, Chauvin M, Gaultier M. Acute digitoxin intoxication treated by intracardiac pacemaker: experience in sixty-eight patients. *Clin Toxicol* 1977; **10**:443–456.

Ekins BR, Watanabe AS. Acute digoxin poisonings: review of therapy. *Am J Hosp Pharm* 1978; **35**:268–277.

Rotmensch HH, Graff E, Terdiman R et al. Furosemide-induced forced diuresis in digoxin intoxication. *Arch Intern Med* 1978; **138**:1495–1497.

Warren SE, Fanestil DD. Digoxin overdose. Limitations of hemoperfusion-hemodialysis treatment. *JAMA* 1979; **242**: 2100–2101.

DISINFECTANTS

General considerations

Serious poisoning with household disinfectants is now uncommon compared with some decades ago when Lysol (50% cresol) was frequently used in suicide attempts. The active constituent of most present-day liquid disinfectants is dichlorometaxylenol (DCMX) though there are still some which contain phenol (carbolic acid) or cresol (methylphenol). In addition they contain miscellaneous other ingredients including soaps, castor oil, isopropanol and pine oil (terpene alcohols) which vary from one brand to another and add significantly to the toxicity when large volumes are ingested. There is considerable knowledge about the toxic effects of phenol and cresol (which for practical purposes are identical). Information about DCMX is very limited but it probably causes similar harm.

Features

Ingestion of large quantities causes burns of the lips, mouth and upper alimentary tract. Not uncommonly spillage on to the face and chest occurs. Initially the lesions are white and become brown in a few days. The burns are said to be painless because of destruction of the nerve endings. Coma may supervene and hypotension, shock and hypothermia are common. A severe metabolic acidosis is usually present and laryngeal oedema, respiratory failure, myocardial damage and renal failure may develop. Aspiration into the lungs produces a haemorrhagic tracheobronchitis and pneumonitis. In rare cases methaemoglobinaemia and intravascular haemolysis have been reported. The urine is usually grey or black in colour and, together with the breath, blood and gastric contents, may smell strongly of phenol.

Treatment

Gastric aspiration and lavage should be carried out provided the airway can be protected. Corticosteroids or, rarely, tracheostomy may be necessary if laryngeal oedema is severe. Metabolic acidosis should be corrected and other supportive measures implemented according to the patient's condition. The possibility that isopropanol is contributing to the clinical picture should be considered and treated appropriately if present (p. 125).

There is extremely little objective information about the value of methods to enhance elimination of absorbed phenols. In one case haemodialysis failed to remove significant quantities of cresol. DCMX is more soluble in alkaline than acid media and alkalinisation of the urine may be worth trying. Plasmapheresis may help since DCMX is concentrated several-fold in red blood cells.

References

Archer LNJ. Upper airways obstruction after Dettol ingestion. *Br Med J* 1979; **2**:19–20.

Cregeen R, Proudfoot AT. Lysol ingestion. In press.

Joubert P, Hundt H, du Toit P. Severe Dettol (chloroxylenol and terpineol) poisoning. *Br Med J* 1978; **1**:890.

Meek D, Piercy DM, Gabriel R. Fatal self-poisoning with Dettol. *Postgrad Med J* 1977; **53**:229–231.

DISOPYRAMIDE

General considerations

Disopyramide is an antidysrhythmic drug which has mild anticholinergic actions and electrophysiological properties similar to quinidine. Only a few cases of accidental and intentional overdosage have been reported to date but most were fatal.

Features

Information on the sequence of events in human poisoning is sketchy but serious effects are often apparent within a short time of ingestion since disopyramide is rapidly and almost completely absorbed. Cyanosis, drowsiness, coma and respiratory and cardiac arrest may occur within 2 hours. Though conventional resuscitative procedures may produce initial improvement, ventricular dysrhythmias and aponea often recur without warning and prove refractory to treatment. Pulmonary oedema is usually present at autopsy. Convulsions were reported in a child who died.

Animal experiments have shown that the primary event in acute disopyramide poisoning is acute circulatory failure with dysrhythmias and respiratory arrest occurring secondarily.

Treatment

The stomach should be emptied if more than the therapeutic dose has been ingested within 4 hours and the blood pressure and cardiac rhythm monitored continuously. A venous line must be established in anticipation of the need for treatment of sudden hypotension or dysrhythmias. Electrolyte and acid-base disturbances should be sought and treated.

Limited experience suggests that isoprenaline is the most effective treatment for bradycardia and hypotension following disopyramide overdosage. The use of related anti-dysrhythmic drugs should be avoided since they may worsen the depression of myocardial contractility. Cardiac pacing may be attempted in the event of isoprenaline failing to achieve an acceptable heart rate and output but the threshold for pacing may be high.

Reference

Holt DW, Helliwell M, O'Keeffe B. Successful management of serious disopyramide poisoning. *Postgrad Med J* 1980; **56**:256–260.

ERGOTAMINE

General considerations

Poisoning with ergotamine tartrate is usually chronic or subacute and due to therapeutic overdosage with anti-migraine preparations. Acute poisoning with a single large dose is rare.

Features

The features of ergotamine poisoning are mainly due to constriction of peripheral arteries. There may be paraesthesiae, numbness, pain and feelings of cold in one or more limbs and the skin is pale or cyanosed with reduced temperature. Digital gangrene may develop in severe poisoning. In subacute cases there may be a history of intermittent claudication and involvement of the renal arteries may present as acute or chronic renal failure. The volume of the peripheral pulses is reduced, or these may be impalpable and the blood pressure is correspondingly low. Consciousness may be impaired after acute overdosage but in some cases this will be due to CNS depressants included in some migraine preparations. Tachycardia, hypotension, raised respiratory rate, haemorrhagic gastritis and cerebral oedema have been reported.

Treatment

The stomach should be emptied if more than ten tablets have been taken during the preceding 4 hours. Analgesics may be required for severe ischaemic pain. Various measures, including vasodilators such as nitroprusside and papaveretum, heparin, sympathetic block and low molecular weight dextran have been used in patients with severe arterial insufficiency but their value is uncertain. Most patients improve with stopping the drug and simple symptomatic measures.

References

Jones EM, Williams B. Two cases of ergotamine poisoning in infants. *Br Med J* 1966; **1**:466.
Pusey CD, Rainford DJ. St Anthony's fire and pseudochronic renal failure. *Br Med J* 1977; **2**:935.

ETHANOL

General considerations

Ethanol (ethyl alcohol) is toxicologically important, not only as a poison in its own right, but because it is ubiquitous and potentiates the CNS depressant effects of other psychotropic drugs. For some years 60–70 per cent of self-poisoning episodes in men and a steadily increasing percentage of those in women (currently about 40 per cent) have been associated with the consumption of alcohol. As a result, clinicians frequently have difficulty in assessing the extent to which the patient's clinical condition is the result of ethanol and how much is due to other drugs taken simultaneously.

Chronic ingestion of excessive quantities of ethanol is also important since it induces the hepatic microsomal oxidase enzyme system, thereby allowing the alcoholic patient to metabolise some drugs more rapidly. This effect may act to advantage when barbiturates are taken in overdosage but is a disadvantage when paracetamol (acetaminophen) is taken.

Ethanol is mainly metabolised in the liver to acetaldehyde and thence to acetate. The reactions are catalysed by alcohol and aldehyde dehydrogenases. Alcohol dehydrogenase is readily saturated and ethanol is removed according to zero-order kinetics at a rate of about 10 ml/h.

Features

Poisoning with ethanol produces varying degrees of CNS depression including coma, hypotension, hypothermia, respiratory failure and death. The breath usually has a characteristic odour and there is an ever-present risk of vomiting, respiratory obstruction and aspiration into the lungs. Arterial blood gas analysis often shows a mild metabolic acidosis and rarely alcohol-induced hypoglycaemia may occur, particularly in children.

Treatment

If large quantities of ethanol have been ingested within 4 hours or consciousness is seriously impaired, the stomach should be emptied provided the airway can be protected. Treatment thereafter is supportive and significant improvement within a few hours can be confidently expected. Head injury should be excluded by careful examination. Ethanol is readily removed by haemodialysis but it is doubtful if this form of treatment should ever be necessary for uncomplicated poisoning.

Intravenous fructose (200 g over 30 min) has also been recommended on the basis of the claim that it increases the rate of metabolism of ethanol by up to 25 per cent. However, not every study has confirmed this benefit. On the other hand there is general agreement that fructose in this dosage causes epigastric and retrosternal discomfort and, more important, exacerbates any pre-existing metabolic acidosis by increasing lactic acid production in the liver. The drawbacks of treatment with fructose outweigh the dubious gains.

Blood ethanol concentrations

Blood ethanol concentrations are most accurately measured by gas–liquid chromatography but few hospital laboratories are able to provide this analysis on an emergency basis. However, breath alcohol analysers have recently been introduced into clinical practice and are scaled to give a result in terms of blood alcohol concentration. They can be used on unconscious as well as conscious patients. While the results are not so accurate, they give a reasonable indication of the magnitude of the ethanol concentration and can be used at the bedside.

Blood ethanol concentrations in poisoned patients vary widely but values up to 3 g/l are commonplace and there are reports of uneventful recovery from concentrations of 6–8 g/l.

References

Levy R, Elo T, Hanenson IB. Intravenous fructose treatment of acute alcohol intoxication. *Arch Intern Med* 1977; **137**:1175–1177.
Ragan FA, Samuels MS, Hite SA. Ethanol ingestion in children. *JAMA* 1979; **242**:2787–2788.

ETHCHLORVYNOL

General considerations

In the United Kingdom the popularity of ethchlorvynol, a tertiary acetylenic alcohol, as a hypnotic has fortunately declined greatly in recent years and poisoning with it is now very uncommon. However, it continues to be used therapeutically and is misused by addicts in North America. Ethchlorvynol is a volatile, brownish liquid with a characteristic pungent smell.

Features

The features of acute poisoning closely resemble those of barbiturate intoxication with depression of consciousness, hyporeflexia, hypotension, hypothermia and respiratory depression. Profound coma is not uncommon and the depth does not usually fluctuate. The main difference from barbiturate poisoning is that the duration of coma due to ethchlorvynol is particularly protracted, commonly lasting four or five days. The potential for serious respiratory complications is increased accordingly.

Severe, non-cardiac, pulmonary oedema may follow the intravenous injection of ethchlorvynol and is due to a direct effect on pulmonary capillaries by the drug itself rather than the vehicle in which it is diluted.

Treatment

The stomach should be emptied if more than ten capsules have been taken within the preceding 4 hours or at any interval after ingestion if the patient is unconscious. Meticulous supportive care is mandatory. The elimination of ethchlorvynol is only very slightly enhanced by haemodialysis, even against soybean oil and it is not recommended. Haemoperfusion is also of limited value because of the large volume of distribution of the drug but may be worth attempting in very severe poisoning.

Pulmonary oedema due to intravenous ethchlorvynol usually clears within 24 hours but oxygen and intermittent positive pressure respiration may be necessary.

References

Benowitz N, Abolin C, Tozer T, et al. Resin hemoperfusion in ethchlorvynol overdose. *Clin Pharmacol Ther* 1980; **27**:236–242.

Glauser FL, Smith WR, Caldwell A, et al. Ethchlorvynol (Placidyl)-induced pulmonary edema. *Ann Intern Med* 1976; **84**:46–48.

Lynn RI, Honig CL, Jatlow PI, Kliger AS. Resin hemoperfusion for treatment of ethchlorvynol overdose. *Ann Intern Med* 1979; **91**:549–553.

ETHYLENE GLYCOL

General considerations

Ethylene glycol is readily available as the major constituent of antifreeze preparations. It has a bitter-sweet taste and may be drunk accidentally by children or intentionally by adults, either for deliberate self-poisoning or as a substitute for alcohol. Most of the serious consequences are thought to be due to its toxic intermediate metabolites, including glycolaldehyde and glycolic, glyoxylic and oxalic acids. Metabolism is catalysed by alcohol dehydrogenase.

Features

The course of ethylene glycol poisoning can be divided into three phases. During the first few hours there is ataxia, slurred speech, nausea, vomiting, occasionally minor haematemesis, convulsions and drowsiness leading to coma. A variety of ocular signs may be present including nystagmus, ophthalmoplegia and, later, papilloedema. The neurological features are most prominent 6–12 hours after ingestion.

The second phase (12–24 hours after ingestion) is dominated by cardio-respiratory problems, the respiratory rate usually being increased with central cyanosis, tachycardia and a slight rise in blood pressure. Cardiac failure and bronchopneumonia may be terminal events in severe cases.

The features of the final phase are due to the onset of renal tubular necrosis with bilateral renal angle and loin pain and oliguria. A diffuse myositis may also be present.

Urine examination usually reveals albuminuria, haematuria and oxalate crystals. A polymorph leukocytosis (up to 40 000/mm³) is common. The plasma potassium is raised and the bicarbonate is frequently < 10 mmol/l due to severe metabolic acidosis. Blood lactate concentrations may be raised while the calcium is reduced by chelation with oxalic acid to form calcium oxalate. Serum creatine phosphokinase may be raised if a myositis is present.

Treatment

The stomach should be emptied if the patient presents within 4 hours of ingestion, taking appropriate steps to protect the airway. Arterial blood gas analysis and measurement of the serum calcium should be requested urgently. Metabolic acidosis should be corrected with intravenous sodium bicarbonate and hypocalcaemia by giving calcium gluconate (10 ml of 10% solution) as necessary. An adequate fluid intake should be ensured and the urine volume must be monitored carefully to detect oliguria at the earliest moment.

The toxicity of ethylene glycol can be reduced by slowing its metabolism by giving sufficient ethanol (5–10 g/h intravenously) to keep the blood ethanol concentration between 1–2 g/l. The ethanol competes with ethylene glycol as a substrate for alcohol dehydrogenase. In severe cases haemodialysis should be used to remove ethylene glycol and may also be necessary for the treatment of renal failure.

References

Scully RE, Galdabini JJ, McNeely BU. Case records of the Massachusetts General Hospital: Case 38–1979. *New Engl J Med* 1979; **301**: 650–657.
Vale JA, Widdop B, Bluett NH. Ethylene glycol poisoning. *Postgrad Med J* 1976; **52**: 598–602.

FLUORIDE

General considerations

Sodium fluoride was formerly used as a rodenticide and insecticide and is still occasionally used for delousing animals. Its most common use now, however, is in very low dosage for prophylaxis against dental caries. Fortunately, in this form (2.2 mg sodium fluoride per tablet) a few hundred tablets would have to be ingested before serious poisoning was likely. Hydrogen fluoride, hydrofluoric acid and its acid salts are used in industry. Systemic fluoride poisoning may occur by ingestion, inhalation or skin contamination. Fluoride is a potent inhibitor of cell metabolism producing effects similar to hypoxia. It also inhibits haemostasis.

Features

The immediate effects of ingestion of inorganic fluorides are nausea, hypersalivation, vomiting and abdominal pain. There may be a soapy taste in the mouth. A haemorrhagic gastroenteritis ensues. Absorbed fluoride ions chelate calcium leading to tetany, hypocalcaemic convulsions and ventricular tachycardia and fibrillation with some victims having as many as fifty or sixty episodes of fibrillation despite antidysrhythmic therapy. Coma occurs due to hypoxia and a direct CNS effect of the fluoride. Respiratory failure and acute renal tubular necrosis may develop. Laboratory investigation confirms hypocalcaemia and there is often a severe metabolic acidosis. The plasma magnesium concentration may also be reduced.

Inhalation of hydrogen fluoride produces laryngeal and pulmonary oedema. Fluoride skin burns are usually deep and exceedingly painful.

Treatment

Ingestion of sodium fluoride in dental caries prophylaxis formulations does not require treatment unless a hundred or more tablets have been taken. It is sufficient to give liberal quantities of milk, the calcium content of which reacts with fluoride to form insoluble calcium fluoride.

If other inorganic fluorides have been taken gastric lavage should be carried out using a weak solution of either calcium hydroxide or calcium chloride. Alternatively, aluminium hydroxide given after gastric lavage will reduce fluoride absorption.

The cardiac rhythm must be monitored continuously and facilities for defibrillation and assisted respiration should be immediately available. Acid-base disturbances and hypocalcaemia should be sought and corrected. Very large quantities of calcium gluconate may be necessary. Frequent measurement of the serum calcium is essential and a good urinary output will promote fluoride excretion. Haemodialysis has occasionally been used to eliminate inorganic fluoride but should rarely be required.

Injection of calcium gluconate around fluoride skin burns reduces the risk of systemic fluoride intoxication but surgical advice about management of the skin ulcers will be required.

Plasma fluoride concentrations

Plasma concentrations of up to 20 mg/l have been reported after acute poisoning but, even without treatment, they fall rapidly as the fluoride is taken up by tissues, particularly bone. Renal fluoride excretion continues at a high rate for several days.

References

Simpson E, Rao LGS, Evans RM, Wilkie W, Rodger JC, Lakhani A. Calcium metabolism in a fatal case of sodium fluoride poisoning. *Ann Clin Biochem* 1980; **17**:10–14.

Spoerke DG, Bennett DL, Gullekson DJK. Toxicity related to acute low dose sodium fluoride ingestions. *J Fam Pract* 1980; **10**:139–140.

GLUTETHIMIDE

General considerations

Glutethimide is a highly lipid-soluble hypnotic which is chemically and pharmacologically similar to barbiturates; it enjoyed widespread popularity in the 1960's but is now much less commonly prescribed. Therapeutic doses induce hepatic microsomal oxidase enzymes and abstinence from regular large doses may precipitate a severe withdrawal syndrome. Glutethimide is metabolised in the liver and one of its metabolites, 4-hydroxy-2-ethyl-2-phenyl glutarimide, is active and thought to account for some of the features of poisoning.

Features

In common with barbiturates, glutethimide overdosage causes profound coma, respiratory depression (less frequently), hypotension, hypothermia and skin blisters. Convulsions may occur. The depth of coma tends to fluctuate and the pupils are commonly dilated, allegedly due to the claimed anticholinergic actions of the drug. There is conflicting evidence that glutethimide poisoning carries the special hazards of sudden apnoea and pulmonary and cerebral oedema. Papilloedema was found in five out of a series of eleven patients who claimed to have taken 12 g or more.

Elevation of serum enzymes has been reported in glutethimide overdosage reflecting skeletal muscle pressure damage.

Treatment

Central nervous system depression is treated conventionally (p. 24) and patients must be constantly observed for early signs of the special risks mentioned above. The stomach should be emptied if more than ten tablets have been ingested or the patient is unconscious. Facilities for endotracheal intubation and assisted ventilation must be immediately available. Cerebral oedema is treated with mannitol and dexamethasone (p. 51) and care should be taken not to overload the patient with intravenous fluid.

Only about 2 per cent of absorbed glutethimide is excreted unchanged in the urine and attempts to enhance elimination by forced diuresis are useless and potentially lethal. Similarly, conventional haemodialysis removes relatively little drug and though the clearance can be increased by using a lipid dialysate such as soyabean oil this procedure has not been shown to have significant therapeutic advantages over intensive supportive care. In rare cases in which there is good reason to eliminate glutethimide as quickly as possible and the appropriate criteria are satisfied (p. 49), charcoal or resin haemoperfusion is the treatment of choice.

Prognosis

Patients may take 48–72 hours or occasionally longer to recover from deep coma caused by glutethimide. While some studies have shown that the mortality from even severe poisoning can be very low, others suggest that it is considerably higher than that of barbiturate overdosage and among the highest of any drug-induced coma.

Plasma glutethimide concentrations

Plasma glutethimide concentrations of up to 60 mg/l are usual in severe poisoning but they do not correlate well with the depth or duration of coma or development of complications. This may be partly due to the unsatisfactory analytical methods in common use. There is very little data using specific methods for glutethimide and its active metabolites.

References

Leading article. Glutethimide—an unsafe alternative to barbiturate hypnotics. *Br Med J* 1976; **1**; 1424.

Koffler A, Bernstein M, LaSette A, Massry SG. Fixed-bed charcoal haemoperfusion. *Arch Intern Med* 1978; **138**: 1691–1694.

HOLLY

General considerations

The attractive red berries of the holly tree, *Ilex aquifolium*, appear around Christmas and are commonly eaten by children. They contain ilexanthin and ilex acid.

Features

Even after eating up to twenty berries the majority of children suffer no ill effects. A few may develop vomiting and diarrhoea.

Treatment

Treatment is usually superfluous. Symptomatic measures may be necessary in a small proportion of cases.

INSULIN

General considerations

Most individuals who deliberately inject themselves with large doses of insulin are insulin-dependent diabetics though occasionally their non-diabetic relatives, and doctors or nurses, may do so. The incidence of self-poisoning with insulin may be higher than the relatively small number of cases reported in the literature would suggest. Virtually every type of insulin has been used for self-poisoning and occasionally for murder.

Features

The patient may be a known diabetic or have evidence of repeated injection over the thighs. It is not uncommon to find an empty syringe and vials by the patient. Examination will reveal the usual signs of hypoglycaemia and the diagnosis may be rapidly confirmed by measurement of the blood glucose concentration and by the clinical response to intravenous glucose. Care must be exercised when interpreting the results of 'stick' tests for estimating blood glucose levels as they may be unreliable.

Frequently the severity of hypoglycaemia is not as marked as might be anticipated from the quantity of insulin injected, suggesting that there is a rate-limiting system for the blood glucose response to plasma insulin which is not affected by major increases in circulating insulin levels. The limited severity of hypoglycaemia after overdosage in some cases may be one of the factors leading to under-detection of this type of self-poisoning.

Brain damage may occur if hypoglycaemia is severe and protracted before treatment is started. Cerebral oedema may occur.

Treatment

If there is any clinical suspicion of hypoglycaemia, whether or not due to insulin overdosage, a venous blood sample should be taken to substantiate the diagnosis and 50 ml of 50% glucose injected intravenously without waiting for the result. Occasionally this dose will have to be repeated before a response is obtained. It is then advisable to establish an intravenous line so that further glucose can be given with ease should hypoglycaemia recur. Hypokalaemia must be corrected. The patient should also be given a carbohydrate-rich meal as soon as he is able to eat. Cerebral oedema should be treated conventionally (p. 51).

Prognosis

The majority of patients make a complete recovery though there is a risk of recurrent hypoglycaemia, depending upon the duration of action of the insulin involved. There is no evidence that acute massive overdosage alters future long-term insulin requirements.

Plasma insulin concentrations

Plasma concentrations of immunoreactive insulin up to 2000 μU/ml have been found after self-poisoning.

Reference

Critchley JAJH, Proudfoot AT. Massive acute insulin overdosage. In press.

IRON

General considerations

Acute iron poisoning is predominantly a childhood problem though adults occasionally ingest large quantities in self-poisoning episodes. There are numerous, probably too numerous, iron preparations on the market and their widespread prescription for anaemia, presumed anaemia and during pregnancy makes them readily available to all age groups including young children. Moreover, the brightly coloured tablets may be indistinguishable from sweets. The incidence of this common and particularly serious childhood poisoning could be reduced by better care of medicines in the home and insistence on the use of child-resistant containers.

Features

The clinical course of acute iron poisoning is traditionally divided into four phases. The first comprises the first few hours after ingestion when vomiting, diarrhoea and abdominal pain are common. The vomitus and stools are usually dark grey or black due to the disintegrating iron preparation but may later become blood-stained due to corrosive effects on the upper gastrointestinal mucosa. The majority of mild poisonings do not progress beyond this point and symptoms settle within 6–8 hours. In severe poisoning first phase features also include drowsiness, coma, convulsions, metabolic acidosis and shock (which is often more severe than would be expected from the amount of gastrointestinal fluid and blood loss). It has been attributed to the effect of circulating free iron (i.e. serum iron in excess of the total iron binding capacity) and release of vasodilator material from the liver. A few patients die in this phase from progressive circulatory failure and coma.

During the second phase, starting 6–12 hours after ingestion, symptoms abate as the iron is taken up by the reticulo-endothelial system. After a lull of 12–48 hours a minority of patients enter the third phase in which there is severe shock, metabolic acidosis, jaundice with its attendant coagulation abnormalities, hypoglycaemia and renal failure. Intestinal infarction has also been reported. The mortality in this phase is high and the liver usually shows hepatocellular necrosis most marked in the periportal regions.

The final phase of iron poisoning is due to gastric stricture formation and pyloric stenosis (alone or in combination) with obstructive symptoms starting after 2–5 weeks.

Serum iron concentrations and assessment of severity of poisoning

Although a straight abdominal X-ray may help substantiate the approximate number of tablets ingested it is customary to assess the severity of poisoning by measuring the serum iron and iron binding capacity as an emergency. Initial serum iron concentrations in poisoned children have been correlated with the presence of shock and/or coma, the generally accepted clinical indices of severe poisoning (Table 4.2).

TABLE 4.2.   Initial serum iron concentrations related to shock and coma in poisoned children.

Initial serum iron (μg/l)	Number in group	Number with coma and/or shock
< 5000	112	9 (8%)
> 5000	46	17 (37%)
> 10000	10	7 (70%)

* Compiled from data given by Westlin WF (1966), *Clin Pediatr* (Phila) 1966; **5**:531.

On the basis of this data it has been recommended that an initial serum iron concentration greater than 5000 µg/l is an indication for energetic treatment with chelating agents. However, several reservations must be noted.

1. The kinetics of iron after acute overdosage in humans have not been adequately investigated but serum concentrations probably peak within 4 hours and fall rapidly thereafter. It follows that the time interval influences the level above which treatment may be necessary. It is thus inappropriate to recommend that a single iron concentration should be an indication for treatment.

2. Interpretation of serum iron levels will be even more difficult when slow-release formulations have been ingested though there is as yet no published evidence on this point.

3. Concern has been expressed about hypotension, anaphylaxis and rashes from desferrioxamine and it is desirable to avoid unnecessary treatment. Table 4.2 shows that over 60 per cent of children with initial serum iron concentrations above 5000 µg/l did not have clinically severe poisoning.

The decision to treat iron poisoning with desferrioxamine requires considerable thought and judgement of the overall situation rather than slavish obedience to an arbitrary iron concentration.

Treatment

Preventing absorption

The stomach should be emptied if > 15 tablets have been ingested within 4 hours and a straight abdominal X-ray will demonstrate whether or not emptying has been complete. It has been recommended that desferrioxamine (2 g powder/litre of water) should be added to the lavage fluid to chelate iron remaining in the stomach and a further 10 g be put down the tube at the end of the procedure. This advice has been criticised on the grounds that desferrioxamine does not usually prevent absorption of the amounts of iron commonly involved in poisoning episodes. Moreover the absorbed iron-desferrioxamine complex (ferrioxamine) may cause serious hypotension and the addition of the recommended quantities of desferrioxamine make satisfactory lavage in adults very costly since large volumes are often needed. Sodium bicarbonate (5%) or disodium phosphate solutions (usually in the form of Fleet enemas—sodium dihydrogen phosphate 16% and trisodium phosphate 6%) diluted 1:4 with water before use are cheaper alternatives. These complex with iron to form the relatively insoluble carbonates and phosphates respectively. It is preferable to use bicarbonate since disodium phosphate may produce life-threatening hypocalcaemia and hyperphosphataemia. 100 ml of 5% sodium bicarbonate should be left in the stomach before the tube is removed.

If a slow-release iron formulation has been ingested and tablets remain in the bowel after gastric lavage the use of whole gut lavage (p. 38) should be considered.

Supportive measures

Arterial blood gas analysis is mandatory in severe iron poisoning and any acid-base disturbance should be corrected. Liver function tests, particularly the prothrombin time ratio, must be monitored at least daily if severe liver damage is suspected. Adequate replacement of fluid and blood losses is essential. Hepatic and renal failure should be managed conventionally.

Specific therapy

Parenteral desferrioxamine is the treatment of choice for severe iron poisoning. It should be given immediately, without waiting for the serum iron concentration, if it is clinically obvious that poisoning is severe (i.e. coma or shock are present). It is usually given intramuscularly (2 g for an adult and 1 g for a child) combined with intravenous infusion at a rate which must not exceed 15 mg/kg/h to avoid hypotension. The total intravenous dose should not exceed 80 mg/kg/24 h. The iron-desferrioxamine complex (ferrioxamine) is excreted in the urine, making it orange-red in colour, and may be eliminated by dialysis if renal failure develops.

Prognosis

Previous estimates indicating a high mortality from acute iron poisoning were almost certainly biased by the tendency to report only severe and fatal cases. The overall mortality is probably much less than 5 per cent but survival from serious poisoning depends upon administration of desferrioxamine at the earliest possible moment.

References

Bachrach L, Correa A, Levin R, Grossman M. Iron poisoning: complications of hypertonic phosphate lavage therapy. *J Pediatr* 1979; **94**: 147–149.

Eriksson F, Johansson SV, Mellstedt H, Strandberg O, Wester PO. Iron intoxication in two adult patients. *Acta Med Scand* 1974; **196**: 231–236.

Gleason WA, de Mello DE, de Castro FJ, Connors JJ. Acute hepatic failure in severe iron poisoning. *J. Pediatr* 1979; **95**: 138–140.

Greenblatt DJ, Allen MD, Koch-Weser J. Accidental iron poisoning in childhood. *Clin Pediatr* (Phila) 1976; **15**: 835–838.

Haddad LM. Iron poisoning, *JACEP* 1976; **5**: 691–693.

Henriksson P, Nilsson L, Nilsson IM, Stenberg P. Fatal iron intoxication with multiple coagulation defects and degradation of factor VIII and factor XIII. *Scand J Haematol* 1979; **22**: 235–240.

Knott LH, Miller RC. Acute iron intoxication with intestinal infarction. *J Pediatr Surg* 1978; **13**: 720–721.

ISONIAZID

General considerations

Acute isoniazid overdosage is uncommon and most recent cases have been reported in American Indians and Eskimos, for whom the drug has been prescribed for the treatment of active tuberculosis or tuberculin convertors. Though most cases are the result of deliberate self-poisoning it has been suggested that others may be attempts to obtain an LSD-type 'trip'.

Isoniazid is acetylated in the liver and individuals may be 'slow' or 'fast' acetylators, the proportion of each varying from one society to another and being genetically determined. The significance of this after massive overdosage has not been investigated. Very little isoniazid is excreted unchanged in the urine.

The mechanism of isoniazid toxicity is not clear but it may act by producing acute pyridoxine (vitamin B_6) deficiency and preventing normal functioning of pyridine nucleotides.

Features

Symptoms usually develop within 2–4 hours. In the early stages hallucinations and visions of brightly-coloured lights have been described but approximately half the patients develop some impairment of consciousness and about 90 per cent have one or more convulsions. Consciousness may not be regained between fits and the patient may remain cyanosed with a tachycardia. There is an ever-present risk of aspiration of gastric contents and respiratory failure. A severe metabolic acidosis is common and is due to raised serum lactate concentrations secondary to hypoxia and convulsions. Hyperpyrexia may also develop.

Hyperglycaemia and a polymorph leukocytosis occur frequently and elevation of serum osmolality, aspartate aminotransferase and lactate dehydrogenase have been noted occasionally. Transient peripheral neuropathy was described in one man treated by haemodialysis.

Treatment

The first priorities are to establish and maintain a patent airway and to control convulsions. The latter may be refractory to conventional measures until large quantities of pyridoxine have been given. Once the patient's condition has stabilised consideration should be given to emptying the stomach. Metabolic acidosis and hypoxia must be corrected.

It has been claimed that the mortality of acute isoniazid poisoning can be considerably reduced by giving large quantities of pyridoxine within the first few hours after ingestion. The recommended dose for an adult is 1 g intravenously for each gram of isoniazid ingested or, if the latter is unknown, 5 g in 50 ml intravenously over 5 minutes and repeated at intervals of 20–30 minutes until convulsions cease and consciousness is regained. If the efficacy of this treatment is confirmed by controlled trials, attempts to enhance the elimination of isoniazid are superfluous. Forced diuresis would not be expected to be beneficial since little drug is excreted unchanged. The value of haemodialysis and haemoperfusion has not been determined.

Prognosis

Prior to the introduction of pyridoxine treatment the mortality of acute isoniazid poisoning varied from 12 to 21 per cent. Adequate, early treatment should make death unlikely.

References

Cameron WM. Isoniazid overdose. *Can Med Assoc J* 1978; **118**:1413–1415.
Bear ES, Hoffman PF, Siegel SR, Randall RE. Suicidal ingestion of

isoniazid: an uncommon cause of metabolic acidosis. *South Med J* 1976; **69**:31–32.

Naranjo G, Lampe KF. Childhood and adolescent poisoning by isoniazid. *Paediatrician* 1977; **6**:271–277.

Miller J, Robinson A, Percy AK. Acute isoniazid poisoning in childhood. *Am J Dis Child* 1980; **134**:290–292.

ISOPROPANOL

General considerations

Isopropanol (isopropyl alcohol) is a constituent of a variety of preparations including disinfectants, solvents, cosmetics and pharmaceutical preparations. In some countries it is available in a 70 per cent solution as a 'rubbing alcohol'. Percutaneous absorption is low but poisoning can readily occur by inhalation. Usually, however, it is the result of ingestion, often by alcoholics seeking a substitute for ethanol. One case of rectal self-administration has been described. Isopropanol is metabolised by alcohol dehydrogenase, the principal metabolite being acetone.

Features

The features of isopropanol intoxication resemble those of ethanol poisoning with loss of consciousness, vasodilatation, hypotension, respiratory depression, hyporeflexia and hypothermia. Patients who become severely hypotensive usually die. The CNS depressant effect of isopropanol is twice that of the same volume of ethanol. Nausea, vomiting and abdominal pain are commoner than with ethanol and a haemorrhagic gastritis may occur. Renal failure, rhabdomyolysis, myoglobinuria, haemolytic anaemia and elevation of the cerebrospinal fluid protein content are rare complications.

Acetone may be detected in the breath, blood and urine.

Treatment

The vast majority of patients require no more than gastric emptying and supportive measures. Haemodialysis readily removes isopropanol and its metabolites and its use should be considered in patients who are desperately ill and have high plasma isopropanol concentrations (see the criteria for haemoperfusion, p. 49).

Plasma isopropanol concentrations

Plasma concentrations up to 5.2 g/l have been reported in severely poisoned patients.

Reference

Agarwal SK. Non-acidotic acetonemia: a syndrome due to isopropyl alcohol intoxication. *J Med Soc NJ* 1979; **76**:914–916.

LABURNUM

General considerations

In Britain laburnum (*Cytisus anagroides*) is probably the most common plant poison encountered in clinical practice. The laburnum tree flowers in the late spring and early summer and for some months bears pods resembling small peas containing up to eight seeds. All parts of the plant, particularly the bark and seeds, are poisonous and it is usually the latter that are involved in childhood poisoning. Cytosine, an alkaloid, is the major toxic agent.

Features

The vast majority of children do not eat enough laburnum seeds to develop symptoms. In rare cases, nausea, vomiting, hypersalivation, drowsiness, incoordination, muscle twitching and convulsions occur. Mydriasis and a tachycardia may be present. Only one death from laburnum poisoning has been recorded in Britain in the last 50 years.

Treatment

Treatment is usually superfluous. It has been suggested that the stomach should be emptied but even this is debatable unless a large number of seeds has been ingested. Routine hospitalisation is unnecessary and it is sufficient to inform parents about the symptoms that can occur and to advise them to bring the child back to hospital should they develop. In these cases supportive care is all that can be offered.

Reference

Forrester RM. Have you eaten laburnum? *Lancet* 1979; **1**:1073.

LEAD

General considerations

In contrast to chronic and sub-acute intoxication, acute lead poisoning is extremely rare. There is one report of five drug addicts who injected themselves intravenously with a solution containing ground-up lead and opium pills.

Features

Abdominal, back and limb pains start soon after injection and are associated with general malaise. Hepatocellular jaundice and hepatic failure may develop a few days later together with oliguria and renal failure due to tubular necrosis. Haemolysis and a rapid fall in haemoglobin may occur. One patient developed extensive peripheral neuropathy which advanced rapidly to involve the respiratory muscles two weeks after exposure. Unexplained hypocalcaemia has been noted.

Treatment

Treatment of acute lead poisoning is predominantly supportive and includes measures to deal with hepatic and renal failure and intravascular haemolysis. Assisted ventilation may be required if serious weakness of the respiratory muscles develops. In all severe cases sodium calciumedetate should be given to enhance lead elimination. The dose is 1 g dissolved in 500 ml 5% dextrose or normal saline given intravenously over 1 hour. Two doses should be given daily for 3–5 days and the total daily dose should not exceed 80 mg/kg for an adult or 70 mg/kg for a child.

Reference

Beattie AD, Briggs JD, Canavan JSF, Doyle D, Mullin PJ, Watson AA. Acute lead poisoning. *Q J Med* 1975; New Series **44**:275–284.

LITHIUM

General considerations

The increasing use of lithium salts for the long-term control of manic-depressive psychosis has been associated with a rise in the number of cases of serious lithium intoxication. Most have occurred since 1963 and are the result of therapeutic overdosage rather than deliberate self-poisoning. This is hardly surprising since the margin between therapeutic and toxic doses is very small. Serum concentrations must be monitored regularly during treatment if toxicity is to be avoided.

Lithium is an alkali metal which is distributed throughout the body water and concentrated in cells although movement across cell membranes is relatively slow. Therapeutic use of lithium may cause thirst or polyuria (independently), renal impairment and (in about 12 per cent of cases) nephrogenic diabetes insipidus. Since lithium is excreted entirely through the kidneys, patients on long-term treatment are particularly vulnerable to reduction of fluid intake (e.g. as a result of intercurrent physical or mental illness or additional psychotropic medication) or increased fluid loss (e.g. fever, vomiting, diarrhoea, diuretic therapy or the development of diabetes insipidus), either of which may precipitate serious lithium intoxication.

Features

The early features of poisoning in patients on long-term therapy are usually nausea, vomiting and diarrhoea. The later major effects are on the brain and neuromuscular system with ataxia, coarse tremor and drowsiness progressing to coma in severe cases. Initially, muscle tone is greatly increased, cog-wheel rigidity may be present and fasciculation and myoclonus are common. The reflexes are correspondingly increased and convulsions may occur. The limbs are often held in hyperextension with an expressionless face and open eyes (so-called 'coma vigile'). Rare complications include acute renal failure and acute diabetes insipidus.

Hypernatraemia and hypokalaemia may be found and the ECG frequently shows non-specific ST depression and T wave inversion but atrioventricular and intraventricular conduction are usually unaffected.

Treatment

If a large overdose has been taken the stomach should be emptied. Patients who are unconscious require supportive measures but increased muscle tone, convulsions and tenacious bronchial secretions may make adequate airway care extremely difficult.

Intravenous fluids are essential to maintain a good urinary output and the nature of the fluids should be determined by the results of urgent measurement of the plasma urea, electrolytes and osmolality. Underlying diabetes insipidus should be strongly suspected if hypernatraemia is present at the outset and in such cases only isotonic dextrose should be given till the plasma sodium and osmolality return to normal. There is a particular risk of hypernatraemia from saline infusions in lithium poisoning. Potassium supplements should be given as required.

Forced diuresis, peritoneal dialysis and haemodialysis have been used in attempts to eliminate circulating lithium but none is entirely satisfactory. The former carries the risk of salt and water overload and is inappropriate when renal function is impaired. It is best reserved for minor poisoning. Clearance of lithium by peritoneal dialysis is no greater than by forced diuresis and it is of little value. Haemodialysis is the most efficient method of removing lithium from the intravascular compartment but rebound increase in serum concentrations (up to 100 per cent) can be expected within a few hours as the plasma re-equilibrates with the intracellular fluid. Haemodialysis must therefore be repeated frequently, allowing serum lithium concentrations to rise between dialyses.

Serum lithium concentrations

Serum lithium concentrations are measured by flame photometry and therapeutic concentrations lie between 0.8 and 1.2 mmol/l. In general, serum concentrations correlate poorly with the clinical severity of lithium poisoning unless the time of ingestion and duration of treatment are considered. Serious toxicity has been reported with 'therapeutic' levels while other patients have shown few ill effects with levels up to 3.7 mmol/l. The tendency to find higher concentrations after deliberate self-poisoning in patients not on previous chronic therapy may be partly explained by slow distribution of the drug to the tissues in the time available since ingestion. Toxic features may appear as serum concentrations are falling.

Prognosis

Recovery from lithium poisoning may take several days because of the slow rate at which lithium can be removed from cells, particularly in the brain. Some patients die from the complications of prolonged coma while serum lithium concentrations may have fallen satisfactorily. The overall mortality in published cases is about 12 per cent.

Survivors may be left with permanent ataxia and choreoathetosis due to damage involving the basal ganglia and cerebellar connections. Nephrogenic diabetes insipidus usually disappears within a few months of stopping lithium treatment but may be permanent in some cases thus creating problems for the future management of their psychiatric illness.

References

Hansen HE, Amdisen A. Lithium intoxication. *Q J Med* 1978; New Series **47**:123–144.
Warick LH. Lithium poisoning. *West J Med* 1979; **130**:259–263.

LYSERGIC ACID DIETHYLAMIDE (LSD)

General considerations

Hospital admissions following acute intoxication with LSD (lysergic acid diethylamide) are less common now than a few years ago. LSD is usually taken by mouth but is occasionally dissolved and snorted for a faster effect. Its mode of action is poorly understood, but the pleasurable effects it produces are well known. Hospital referral usually results from an acute panic reaction, a schizophrenic-like psychotic state, aggressive outbursts or, rarely, attempts at suicide or homicide.

Features

The features are usually the result of adverse reactions to 'normal' doses. The individual may be found wandering in a confused, agitated state and usually has visual hallucinations. Some patients may be wildly excited and unmanageable. Dilatation of the pupils and mild hypertension are common and occasionally body temperature is raised.

Only a few cases of massive LSD overdosage have been reported. Coma, respiratory arrest and metabolic acidosis are the dominant features. Platelet dysfunction may cause a mild generalised bleeding tendency and polymorph leukocytosis is common.

Treatment

Most patients only require reassurance and sedation. One dose of chlorpromazine (50–100 mg intramuscularly) is usually adequate and preferable to diazepam. If the individual is unconscious the usual supportive measures should be taken.

Prognosis

Recovery is usually complete within a few hours although in some cases hallucinations may persist up to 48 hours and the psychotic state for 3–4 days. Even patients who had serious physical consequences after massive overdosage returned to normal within 12 hours. Flashbacks (brief recurrences of some components of the LSD 'trip') may occur unpredictably up to a year later.

References

Forrest JAH, Tarala RA. 66 hospital admissions due to reactions to lysergide (LSD). *Lancet* 1973; **2**: 1310–1313.
Griggs EA, Ward M. LSD toxicity: a suspected cause of death. *J Ky Med Assoc* 1977; **75**: 172–173.
Klock JC, Boerner U, Becker CE. Coma, hypothermia and bleeding associated with massive LSD overdose. *West J Med* 1974; **120**: 183–188.

LUPIN

General considerations

Lupins (*Lupinus* species) are widely cultivated as garden plants although in some countries there are wild varieties. Their toxicity varies from year to year depending on the conditions of cultivation and some non-poisonous types are used for food. However all parts of the plant, particularly the seeds, may contain toxic alkaloids (mainly of the quinolizidine group) which are not altered by drying.

Lupin seeds are most likely to be ingested by small children.

Features

It is uncommon for enough seeds to be eaten to cause symptoms but large numbers rarely cause convulsions, respiratory depression, muscular weakness and bradycardia. On the other hand there is a recent report of short-lived anticholinergic features (p. 65).

Treatment

Most cases will not require treatment. The stomach should be emptied if large numbers of seeds (>25) have been ingested. Treatment thereafter is symptomatic.

MEFENAMIC ACID

General considerations

The incidence of overdosage (accidental and deliberate) with this widely prescribed analgesic is increasing in Britain.

Features

Convulsions are the most serious feature and occur in 10–20 per cent of patients. They are usually brief and do not recur. Less commonly, vomiting and diarrhoea may develop.

Treatment

The stomach should be emptied if more than twenty capsules or tablets have been ingested within 4 hours. There is no specific treatment. Diazepam may be required for repeated convulsions but otherwise symptomatic measures are rarely required. Complete recovery can be expected within 12 hours.

Plasma mefenamic acid concentrations

Plasma mefenamic acid concentrations of up to 210 mg/l have been reported after overdosage (therapeutic concentrations approx 10 mg/l). Convulsions are most likely to occur in patients with highest concentrations. The plasma half-life, even after overdosage, is very short (2–3 hours).

Reference

Balali-Mood M, Critchley JAJH, Proudfoot AT, Prescott LF. Mefenamic acid overdosage. *Lancet* 1981; **1**: 1354–1356.

MEPROBAMATE

General considerations

Meprobamate enjoyed considerable popularity as a tranquilliser in the 1950's and 1960's, before it was ousted by the benzodiazepines. Acute overdosage with meprobamate was never as common as with barbiturates and non-barbiturate hypnotics. However, meprobamate shares many of the pharmacological properties of barbiturates. Regular use induces hepatic microsomal enzymes and tolerance and acute withdrawal from large doses (>2 g/day) results in an abstinence syndrome. The plasma half-life of meprobamate is about 15 hours.

Features

The features of acute meprobamate poisoning are the same as those of barbiturate overdosage (p. 70). In uncomplicated cases coma seldom lasts longer than 36 hours though occasional deaths have been recorded.

Treatment

The majority of patients require no more than supportive care. The stomach should be emptied if more than fifteen tablets have been ingested in the preceding 4 hours or if the patient is in coma.

Measures to increase elimination of meprobamate are only indicated when urgent recovery of consciousness is desirable or the patient is very severely poisoned. There is no merit in attempting forced diuresis. Haemodialysis removes significant amounts of meprobamate but charcoal haemoperfusion is even more efficient and is preferred. Patients should satisfy the criteria on p. 49 before these techniques are used.

Plasma meprobamate concentrations

Plasma meprobamate concentrations must be measured by a specific method such as gas chromatography. Non-tolerant patients would be expected to be unconscious with levels exceeding 50 mg/l though values of up to 300 mg/l may be encountered after acute poisoning.

References

Crome P, Higgenbottom T, Elliott JA. Severe meprobamate poisoning: successful treatment with haemoperfusion. *Postgrad Med J* 1977: **53**:698–699.

Hoy WE, Marin MG, Rieders F. Resin Hemoperfusion for treatment of a massive meprobamate overdose. *Ann Intern Med* 1980; **93**:455–456.

MERCURY (INORGANIC)

General considerations

Acute inorganic mercury poisoning has occurred after ingestion of mercury salts, particularly mercuric chloride, accidental and deliberate injection of metallic mercury, inhalation of mercury vapour when thermometers or barometers have broken in heated ovens and inhalation of metallic mercury from ruptured bougie bags. Fortunately, the commonest accidental exposure to mercury, the ingestion of the bulbs of clinical thermometers by children, does not lead to poisoning since insignificant quantities are absorbed from the gastrointestinal tract.

Features

The features of inorganic mercury poisoning depend to some extent on the route of exposure.

Ingestion of a single large dose of mercurous chloride (calomel) does not usually cause symptoms since it is poorly absorbed. In contrast the gastrointestinal effects of mercuric chloride have earned this salt the name 'corrosive sublimate'. It produces a corrosive haemorrhagic gastroenteritis with severe vomiting and profuse watery diarrhoea (both of which may contain blood) associated with abdominal cramps, limb muscle pain and shock. Acute renal failure due to a direct effect of mercury on the renal tubule is invariable with severe poisoning.

Inhalation of air containing high mercury vapour concentrations produces symptoms within an hour including cough, chest pain, breathlessness due to an acute pneumonitis, shivering, generalised weakness, anorexia and joint pains. Less acute exposure by the same route leads to nausea, salivation, headache, irritability, fatigue, memory impairment, sleeplessness and incoordination in the upper limbs, the usual features of chronic mercurialism.

An acute inflammatory reaction occurs at the site of subcutaneous injection of metallic mercury but the degree of systemic toxicity is variable. Some patients have no features of poisoning while others become febrile, have muscular spasms, stomatitis, abdominal pain, and progress to renal failure and death. Embolisation of mercury to the lungs may complicate subcutaneous as well as intravenous injection of metallic mercury. Symptoms following the latter also vary.

Inhaled globules of mercury are usually walled off by granulomatous tissue.

Treatment

Treatment for swallowed broken thermometer bulbs is unnecessary.

Patients seen within a few hours of ingestion of mercuric chloride should have a cautious gastric lavage and fluid and blood replaced as necessary. Fluid balance must be carefully monitored and renal failure treated conventionally. Analgesics may be required for pain.

Individuals should be evacuated immediately if the atmosphere is contaminated by mercury vapour.

Surgical excision of subcutaneous metallic mercury should be undertaken to minimise both the local reaction and the risk of systemic poisoning. The completeness of drainage is readily assessed radiologically.

Chelation therapy should be given promptly when features of systemic poisoning develop, regardless of the route of exposure. The drug of choice is dimercaprol (British Anti-Lewisite, BAL) in a maximum dose of 4 mg/kg 4-hourly for two days followed by 3 mg/kg twice daily for 8 days. Penicillamine may also be of value though its role in acute mercury poisoning has not been assessed.

References

Ambre JJ, Welsh MJ, Svare CW. Intravenous elemental mercury injection: blood levels and excretion of mercury. *Ann Intern Med* 1977; **87**:451–453.

Dzau VJ, Szabo S, Chang YC. Aspiration of metallic mercury. *JAMA* 1977; **238**:1531–1532.

Hannigan BG. Self-administration of metallic mercury by intravenous injection. *Br Med J* 1978; **2**:933.

Krohn IT, Solof A, Mobini J, Wagner DK. Subcutaneous injection of metallic mercury. *JAMA* 1980; **243**:548–549.

Sexton DJ et al. A nonoccupational outbreak of inorganic mercury vapor poisoning. *Arch Environ Health* 1978; **33**:186–191.

METALDEHYDE

General considerations

Metaldehyde (metacetaldehyde) is widely available to the public in the form of pellets used for killing slugs. Less frequently it is used as a solid fuel. It is poorly soluble in water.

Features

Small children and animals are most at risk from accidental poisoning but this is rarely serious.

Nausea, vomiting, abdominal pain and diarrhoea often occur after a latent period of 1–3 hours. Severe poisoning is associated with a generalised increase in muscle tone, convulsions, impairment of consciousness and metabolic acidosis. Features of hepatic and renal tubular necrosis may become apparent after 2–3 days.

Treatment

The stomach should be emptied if pellets have been ingested within 4 hours. Treatment thereafter is symptomatic including protection of the airway, control of convulsions and correction of the acid-base disturbance.

METHANOL

General considerations

Methanol (methyl or wood alcohol) is widely used in industry and laboratories as a solvent and is present in toxicologically insignificant concentrations (5%) in methylated and surgical spirits which are comprised mainly of ethanol. It is also used as a windscreen washer fluid. Although poisoning may occur from inhalation of methanol fumes or percutaneous absorption, ingestion is by far the commonest route. Many isolated cases of methanol self-poisoning occur in people who have access to the chemical at work but several epidemics have been reported when illicit alcohol has been adulterated with methanol, or methanol has been taken as an ethanol substitute.

Methanol is metabolised mainly in the liver by alcohol and acetaldehyde dehydrogenases to formaldehyde and formic acid. The rate of metabolism is independent of the plasma concentration and is only about one-seventh as rapid as that of ethanol. The toxicity of methanol is due to its metabolites rather than the parent compound.

Features

Because of the slow rate of production of formaldehyde and formic acid there is frequently a latent period of about 12 hours between ingestion and the onset of symptoms although occasionally the delay may be as long as 72 hours.

Conscious patients complain of headache, weakness, breathlessness and visual symptoms (usually dim or blurred vision and flashing lights). Violent attacks of abdominal colic are common and nausea and vomiting occur in about 50 per cent of cases. Only a minority develop diarrhoea.

The patient often appears pale, apprehensive and restless. Sweating is common but the pulse rate and blood pressure are seldom abnormal till late in the course of the poisoning. Some pass through a phase of excitement before drowsiness and coma supervene. Convulsions occasionally occur.

Visual acuity may be reduced to perception of light or complete blindness. The pupils are usually dilated and unresponsive to light. Hyperaemia of the optic disc is the commonest abnormality on retinoscopy in the acute stage and subsides over 2–7 days.

Peripapillary oedema often occurs but it develops more slowly and persists longer (up to 8 weeks). Venous engorgement and retinal haemorrhages are uncommon.

The abdomen is often rigid. Severe metabolic acidosis is common but Kussmaul's respiration is found in only 25 per cent of cases. Bradycardia is a concomitant of respiratory failure and death follows progressive reduction of cardiac output, respiratory rate and tidal volume.

Cerebral oedema, necrosis in the putamen and haemorrhagic pancreatitis may be found at autopsy.

Plasma methanol concentrations

Diagnosis of acute methanol poisoning in the absence of an adequate history requires a high index of suspicion and if the combination of clinical and acid-base abnormalities raise the possibility, urgent steps should be taken to identify and quantify methanol in plasma. This usually entails having facilities for gas–liquid chromatography. Plasma methanol concentrations in excess of 5000 mg/l have been reported.

Treatment

The stomach should be emptied if more than 20 ml of methanol has been ingested or if the patient is unconscious. Arterial blood gas analysis and correction of metabolic acidosis with intravenous sodium bicarbonate is essential. Convulsions should be controlled with diazepam.

As in ethylene glycol poisoning, ethanol should be given to compete with methanol as a substrate for alcohol dehydrogenase, thereby reducing the rate of formation of formaldehyde and formic acid. Oral treatment (0.5 mg/kg of absolute alcohol followed by 0.25 ml/kg 2-hourly) is only appropriate for minor intoxication. In severe poisoning it should always be given intravenously (5–10 g/h) the rate being adjusted to achieve a plasma ethanol concentration of 1–2 g/l. Treatment must be maintained until the plasma methanol concentration is less than about 200 mg/l.

Haemodialysis removes methanol and its metabolites and, if started early enough, may prevent death and permanent visual damage. The indications for dialysis are ill-defined but it should be considered if the plasma methanol concentration exceeds 500 mg/l, if there is significant metabolic acidosis, or if mental or visual symptoms attributable to the poison are present. Dialysis should be continued till the plasma concentration falls below 250 mg/l.

Prognosis

Severe methanol poisoning is frequently fatal and bradycardia, hypotension and severe acidosis are poor prognostic signs. The commonest long-term sequel is visual impairment, usually central scotomata or complete blindness secondary to optic atrophy. Patients who have gross visual symptoms or signs on presentation are unlikely to improve. Prevention of ocular damage depends on prompt treatment to remove methanol and, more importantly, its toxic metabolites.

References

Dethlefs R, Naraqi S. Ocular manifestations and complications of acute methyl alcohol intoxication. *Med J Aust* 1978; **2**:483–485.

Kahn A, Blum D. Methyl alcohol poisoning in an 8-month-old boy: an unusual route of intoxication. *J. Pediatr* 1979; **94**:841–843.

McCoy HG, Cipolle RJ, Ehlers SM, Sawchuk RJ, Zaske DE. Severe methanol poisoning. Application of a pharmacokinetic model for ethanol therapy and hemodialysis. *Am J Med* 1979; **67**:804–807.

McMartin KE, Ambre JJ, Tephly TR. Methanol poisoning in human subjects. Role for formic acid accumulation in the metabolic acidosis. *Am J Med* 1980; **68**:414–418.

METHAQUALONE

General considerations

Methaqualone is a non-barbiturate hypnotic which is available on its own (Melsed, Quaalude) or in combination with diphenhydramine (Mandrax). Like barbiturates it induces hepatic microsomal enzymes, tolerance and physical dependence. Convulsions and delirium may occur if large doses are withdrawn abruptly. It has been extensively misused by addicts but its poor solubility in water has prevented it being mainlined. In Britain, methaqualone is a Class C controlled drug in the terms of the Misuse of Drugs Act, 1972. The incidence of self-poisoning with this drug has declined considerably in recent years.

Features

The features of methaqualone overdosage are similar whether or not it is taken in combination with diphenhydramine. Coma is common but is seldom as deep as grade 4. Characteristically, muscle tone is increased with hyperreflexia and extensor plantar responses. Myoclonus is commonly present. While respiratory depression is less frequent than with barbiturate poisoning, the incidence of cardiovascular complication is greater. Hypotension, pulmonary oedema and myocardial infarction have been reported. Other less common features include skin blisters, convulsions and bleeding. Peripheral neuropathy has been described in one man after recovery.

Treatment

The stomach should be emptied if the patient is unconscious or more than fifteen tablets have been ingested within 4 hours.

The vast majority of patients recover uneventfully with supportive measures alone. Forced diuresis is useless and is contraindicated by the tendency to pulmonary oedema. Peritoneal dialysis and haemodialysis are of little value, even when plasma methaqualone concentrations are very high. Charcoal haemoperfusion is the best treatment in very severely poisoned patients and if urgent recovery of consciousness is necessary. The criteria outlined on p. 49 must, of course, be satisfied.

Plasma methaqualone concentrations

In general, plasma methaqualone concentrations correlate poorly with depth of coma although values of 10–30 mg/l may be expected with grade 2 or 3 coma and 35–45 mg/l with grade 4 coma. Plasma concentrations at any level of coma will be less in the presence of alcohol or other CNS depressant drugs.

References

Brown SS, Goenechea S. Methaqualone: metabolic, kinetic and clinical pharmacologic observations. *Clin Pharmacol Ther* 1973; **14**; 314–324.
Oh TE, Gordon TP, Burden PW. Unilateral pulmonary oedema and 'Mandrax' poisoning. *Anaesthesia* 1978; **33**: 719–721.

METOCLOPRAMIDE

General considerations

Serious problems with metoclopramide overdosage have not been reported. However the drug not infrequently causes adverse reactions which patients find particularly frightening and doctors find perplexing.

Features

The typical patient is a young woman who has been prescribed metoclopramide for hyperemesis gravidarum. The presenting feature of toxicity is a dystonic reaction, usually in the form of uncontrollable chewing movements of the mouth and tongue, spasmodic torticollis or oculogyric crises. Consciousness is not impaired.

Treatment

Obviously no further metoclopramide should be given. The patient should be reassured and dystonic reactions can be abolished within a few minutes by giving benztropine (2 mg intramuscularly) or orphenadrine (40 mg intramuscularly).

Reference

Low LCK, Goel KM. Metoclopramide poisoning in children. *Arch Dis Child* 1980; **55**: 310–312.

MIANSERIN

General considerations

Mianserin is a tetracyclic antidepressant which has only recently been introduced into clinical practice. It lacks the anticholinergic properties of tricyclic antidepressants and maprotiline. To date, information on acute mianserin overdosage is scanty.

Features

Drowsiness has been the most common feature in poisoned adults but the few patients reported to have been unconscious had taken additional CNS depressants. Hypertension has been found as frequently as hypotension and though dysrhythmias have not been detected, one patient had first degree heart block which reverted to normal as the plasma mianserin concentration fell. In contrast to overdosage with tricyclic antidepressants and maprotiline, convulsions have not yet been reported with mianserin poisoning although the drug may have epileptogenic properties.

Treatment

There is probably no need to empty the stomach unless more than 20 tablets have been taken within 4 hours. Treatment is symptomatic and supportive. Haemodialysis was used to treat one patient who had a plasma mianserin concentration of 780 µg/l 5 hours after ingestion but it failed to alter the rate of elimination of the drug and was obviously ineffective.

Plasma mianserin concentrations

Plasma mianserin concentrations in therapeutic doses lie between 30 and 120 µg/l. Concentrations up to 780 µg/l have been reported after overdosage but the data are insufficient for correlation with clinical features.

References

Crome P, Newman B. Poisoning with maprotiline and mianserin. *Br Med J* 1977; **2**: 260.
Green SDR, Kendall-Taylor P. Heart block in mianserin hydrochloride overdose. *Br Med J* 1977; **2**: 1190.

MISTLETOE

General considerations

It is not uncommon for young children to eat mistletoe (*Viscum album*) berries. The toxic principles are known as viscotoxins and are long-chain polypeptides. At least three have been identified and shown to be structurally and pharmacologically similar to the cardiotoxin of cobra venom. They produce progressive depolarisation of muscle cell membranes, perhaps by binding to membrane sites normally occupied by calcium.

Features

Though the potential for serious poisoning is considerable, children seldom eat sufficient berries to develop symptoms. Vomiting, abdominal pain and diarrhoea are the commonest features amongst those who do. Very rarely there may be muscle weakness, bradycardia and circulatory failure.

Treatment

The stomach should be emptied if ten or more berries have been eaten. Treatment will not be required for the vast majority of cases and the remainder are unlikely to require more than symptomatic measures. Calcium gluconate may be worth trying if circulatory failure develops since calcium has been shown experimentally to reverse the effects of viscotoxins on muscle cells.

Reference

Moore HW. Mistletoe poisoning. *J SC Med Assoc* 1963; **59**: 269–271.

MONOAMINE OXIDASE INHIBITORS

Nialamide
Phenelzine
Tranylcypromine

General considerations

Acute overdosage with monoamine oxidase inhibitors is uncommon but the consequences are frequently serious or even fatal. The features of poisoning are due to secondary tissue accumulation of catecholamines rather than to a direct toxic effect of the drug.

Features

There is commonly a latent period of 6–12 hours before tissue catecholamine concentrations increase sufficiently to cause toxicity.

Most features are the result of CNS overactivity. Initially there is a feeling of unease followed by increasing agitation, hallucinations and restlessness. Motor activity may increase to such an extent that the patient performs 'continuous gymnastics' with writhing of the limbs and trunk, grimacing and grinding of the teeth. There is usually associated dilatation of the pupils, nystagmus, tachycardia, rise in blood pressure and profuse sweating. Muscle tone and reflexes are exaggerated with extensor plantar responses. Myoclonus and convulsions are common. Marked pyrexia, disproportionate to the degree of muscular activity, may be present.

Treatment

The stomach should be emptied if ten tablets or more have been ingested within 4 hours. It is advisable to observe any patient who has taken an overdose of monoamine oxidase inhibitors for a minimum of 12 hours for the onset of toxic features.

Treatment is mainly supportive. Haloperidol or chlorpromazine may help reduce overactivity and though there are no reports of the use of beta-adrenergic blockers in this type of poisoning they should be effective if given in large enough doses. Tepid sponging or ice-packs may be required to prevent fever reaching dangerous heights. If convulsions are frequent, curarisation and assisted ventilation may be more appropriate than administration of anticonvulsants.

It has been claimed that haemodialysis is effective but laboratory evidence to support this has not been presented.

References

Ciocatto E, Fagiano G, Bava GL. Clinical features and treatment of overdosage of monoamine oxidase inhibitors and their interaction with other psychotropic drugs. *Resuscitation* 1972; **1**: 69–72.

Matell G, Thorstrand C. A case of fatal nialamid poisoning. *Acta Med Scand* 1967; **181**:79–82.

Matter BJ, Donat PE, Brill ML, Ginn HE. Tranylcypromine sulfate poisoning. *Arch Intern Med* 1965; **116**: 18–20.

Reid DD, Kerr WC. Phenelzine poisoning responding to phenothiazine. *Med J Aust* 1969; **2**: 1214–1215.

MUSHROOMS

General considerations

Of the numerous known genera of fungi it is estimated that some 50 are harmful to man, although about 90 per cent of fatalities are due to one variety, *Amanita phalloides* (the death cap mushroom). The distribution of individual species of fungi varies considerably from one country to another and even within any given country depending on its growth requirements. The constituent toxins may also vary to some extent.

Present-day concern about mushroom poisoning arises from the increasing trend to pick and eat wild varieties as part of the vogue for a return to a more 'natural' diet and the ingestion of hallucinogenic species for 'kicks'. However, the differentiation of poisonous from edible types is not nearly as easy as some suggest and the optimal number of mushrooms necessary for a 'trip' is very much a matter of trial and error. Inevitably some individuals become poisoned. Since doctors will seldom be any wiser in matters of identification than most of their patients it is fortunate that the number of fungi which cause serious illness is so small and that the nature of their toxins and the type and time course of the symptoms they produce are reasonably well-defined. In most cases, however, the mechanisms of toxicity are not known.

When taking the history from someone poisoned with mushrooms attention should be paid to:

1. The interval between ingestion and onset of symptoms, which is crucial in distinguishing between non-serious and potentially fatal poisoning.
2. The number of different varieties of mushrooms eaten. This is important because edible and poisonous types often grow in close proximity.
3. Whether or not alcohol was drunk between eating the mushrooms and the onset of symptoms.
4. Whether or not the fungi were cooked before eating. Some toxins (e.g. haemolysins and some gastrointestinal irritants) are inactivated by heat while others (particularly those with more serious effects) are thermostable.

If possible specimens of the mushrooms should be identified by an expert mycologist.

Features

It is diagnostically and prognostically most valuable to consider the initial features in relation to the time interval since ingestion, as shown in Table 4.3. In general, the sooner symptoms start, the less serious the poisoning although this may not be the case if a mixture of species has been ingested.

Gastrointestinal irritation of early onset usually lasts only a few hours and is seldom severe enough to cause serious dehydration except occasionally in small children. Similarly visual hallucinations do not usually persist longer than 4–6 hours but there are reports of some patients having distortion of perception lasting several days or psychiatric symptoms for weeks.

In mild cases of *Gyromitra* poisoning symptoms usually settle over six days but acute hepatocellular necrosis with its potentially lethal complications may develop in severe cases.

By far the most serious mushroom poisoning is that caused by *Amanita phalloides* and the related species *A. verna* and *A. virosa*. After a latent period of about 12 hours there is usually nausea, severe vomiting and profuse watery diarrhoea comparable to that seen in cholera. These features may subside gradually over several hours and a phase of apparent recovery lasting up to 48–72 hours after ingestion ensues. Evidence of massive hepatic necrosis may then appear and acute renal failure may also develop. The mortality in this phase is high.

Coprine, the toxic principle of the common ink cap, is converted in the body to l-aminocyclopropanol which inhibits alcohol dehydrogenase. Ingestion of alcohol then causes accumulation of acetaldehyde and symptoms identical to the alcohol-disulfiram reaction.

Treatment

The stomach should be emptied if the patient presents within 4 hours unless identification of the mushrooms or the nature of the symptoms indicate that poisoning is mild and is unlikely to become worse.

The majority of patients with early symptoms will not require specific measures but, if severe, appropriate treatment should be given as indicated in Table 4.3.

When hepatotoxic and nephrotoxic species have been ingested, careful monitoring of liver and renal function is mandatory as in

Interval	Initial features	Toxins	Fungi	Treatment for severe symptoms
2 h or less	Nausea, vomiting, diarrhoea	Undetermined gastrointestinal irritants	Numerous fungi including *Entoloma sinuatum*, *Boletus satanas*, *Nalonea sericea*, *Paxillus involutus*, *Agaricus xanthedermus*, *Russula* species, *Tricholoma* species among others	Antiemetics, intravenous fluids, correction of electrolyte imbalance
	Profuse sweating, salivation, vomiting, abdominal colic, diarrhoea, rhinorrhoea, blurred vision	Muscarine	Species of *Clitocybe* and *Inocybe*	Atropine
	Hallucinations without impairment of consciousness	Psilocybin Psilocin	Species of *Psilocybe* and *Panaeolus* including the liberty cap (*Psilocybe semilanceata*)	Reassurance and sedation with diazepam or chlorpromazine
	Hallucinations with impaired consciousness	Ibotenic acid Muscimol	*Amanita muscaria* (fly agaric) and *A. pantherina* (panther cap)	
6 h or more	Very sudden onset headache, dizziness, tiredness, abdominal pain, vomiting	Gyromitrin (hydrolyses to monomethylhydrazine)	*Gyromitra esculenta* (brain fungus)*	See text
12 h (approx)	Severe vomiting, abdominal cramp, profuse watery diarrhoea	Amanitins (cyclic octapeptides)	*Amanita phalloides* (death cap), *A. verna*, *A. virosa* and some species of *Galerina*	See text
Up to 24 h	Flushing, sweating, nausea immediately after alcohol consumption	Coprine (active form l-aminocyclopropanol)	*Coprinus atramentarius* (common ink cap)	Propranolol
72 h or more	Thirst, polyuria leading to renal failure	Unspecified polypeptides	*Cortinarius* species†	Conventional measures for renal failure

*Poisoning and deaths reported mainly from Eastern Europe, particularly Poland.
†Poisoning reported only from Poland, Scotland and Finland.

paracetamol poisoning (p. 162) and prophylactic measures against hepatic encephalopathy should be instituted on the earliest evidence of hepatic damage. In the early stages adequate replacement of fluid and electrolytes lost by vomiting and diarrhoea is essential and anti-emetics such as metoclopramide (10 mg intramuscularly) may be helpful.

The more specific treatment of *A. phalloides*-type poisoning is a matter of considerable debate. Most of the support for particular forms of treatment is anecdotal rather than objective and is, no doubt, in large part due to the difficulty of predicting the outcome without treatment in individual cases. Regular oral activated charcoal has been recommended to interrupt entero-hepatic circu-lation of the toxins and at least has the merit of being harmless, even if it is not of proven efficacy. A variety of drugs including penicillin, phenylbutazone and sulphamethoxazole are thought to increase urinary excretion of amanitins by displacing them from plasma protein binding sites.

Not surprisingly, exchange transfusion, haemodialysis and, more recently, charcoal haemoperfusion have been tried but there is no objective evidence that they remove toxin or improve the prognosis. Apparent reduction of mortality in treated compared with untreated groups is unsatifactory evidence that survival was due to the treatment if the groups cannot be shown to have been similarly poisoned in the first place. *In vitro* experiments suggest that amanitins are poorly dialysable and animal studies indicate that they cannot be detected in the plasma 5 hours after an intravenous dose, having been taken up by tissues or excreted in the urine during that time. Clearly measures aimed at increasing elimination would have to be implemented at a very early stage if there was to be any hope of removing significant quantities.

Another approach has been to try to protect hepatocytes against the toxic effects of amanitins by giving cytochrome C and thioctic acid but, while there is experimental support for their use, their mode of action is far from clear and the results in clinical practice are open to the same criticisms as were directed at methods to increase elimination. Until the matter is clarified, it would seem wise to place most reliance on meticulous supportive care of the patient with acute hepatic necrosis. Should thioctic acid treatment be thought desirable the dose is 25 mg four times daily by intravenous infusion in dextrose on the first day increasing to 75 mg four times daily on the second day if there is evidence of hepatic damage.

References

Becker CE, Tong TG, Boerner U, et al. Diagnosis and treatment of *Amanita phalloides*-type mushroom poisoning. *West J Med* 1976; **125**: 100–109.

Benjamin C. Persistent psychiatric symptoms after eating psilocybin mushrooms. *Br Med J* 1979; **1**: 1319–1320.

Caley MJ, Clark RA. Cardiac arrhythmia after mushroom ingestion. *Br Med J* 1977; **2**: 1633.

Cooles P. Abuse of the mushroom *Panaeolus foenisecii*. *Br Med J* 1980; **280**: 446–447.

Faulstich H. New aspects of *Amanita* poisoning. *Klin Wochenschr* 1979; **57**: 1143–1152.

Giusti GV, Carnevale A. A case of fatal poisoning by *Gyromitra esculenta*. *Arch Toxicol* 1974; **33**: 49–54.

McCormick DJ, Avbel AJ, Gibbons RB. Non-lethal mushroom poisoning. *Ann Intern Med* 1979; **90**: 332–335.

Short AIK, Watling R, MacDonald M, Robson JS. Poisoning by *Cortinarius speciosissimus*. *Lancet* 1980; **2**: 942–944.

NARCOTIC ANALGESICS

Codeine	Etorphine	Oxymorphone
Dextromoramide	Heroin (diacetylmorphine)	Papaveretum
Dextropropoxyphene	Hydromorphone	Pentazocine
Dihydrocodeine	Methadone	Phenazocine
Diphenoxylate	Morphine	Pethidine
Dipipanone	Opium	(meperidine)

General considerations

Opium is derived from the milky fluid which exudes from the cut surface of unripe seed-capsules of *Papaver somniferum*. It contains a number of alkaloids of which the phenanthrene compounds, morphine and codeine, are the most important. Over the years a number of related narcotic drugs have been derived from these or synthesised. They are extensively used as potent analgesics, euphoriants, anti-tussives and anti-diarrhoeal agents.

Codeine is a constituent of many over-the-counter analgesics commonly taken in overdosage but its effects, if any, are completely overshadowed by those of salicylates or paracetamol, the major constituents of such preparations. In Britain dextropropoxyphene is undoubtedly the commonest agent responsible for serious narcotic poisoning. This is due to the recent marked increase in the incidence of self-poisoning with Distalgesic (dextropropoxyphene and para-cetamol). Propoxyphene poisoning has been recognised as a problem in the United States for some years.

Poisoning with narcotics such as morphine, heroin and methadone is usually the result of accidental intravenous overdosage by drug addicts due to the unpredictable potency of 'street' drugs. There are therefore likely to be marked differences in the incidence of this type of narcotic poisoning, being a much larger problem in selected quarters of large cities than in rural areas. Dextromoramide, dipipanone, and dihydrocodeine are also popular with addicts and it seems likely that many doctors who prescribe these drugs do not appreciate that they are narcotic analgesics with the same potential for misuse as morphine and heroin. Prolonged use induces tolerance and profound psychological and physical dependence.

Poisoning with other narcotic analgesics is infrequent but two merit special mention. Diphenoxylate overdosage is not uncommon among children who eat Lomotil tablets (diphenoxylate and atropine) prescribed for treatment of diarrhoea. Etorphine is about 400 times more potent than morphine in man and is used in veterinary medicine for immobilising large animals. Severe poisoning from both accidental and deliberate self-injection has been reported.

Features

Coma, pinpoint pupils and marked reduction of the respiratory rate are the hallmarks of poisoning with narcotic analgesics. The depth of respiration may also be reduced but in some cases it may seem normal or even increased. Respiratory arrest, hypotension and hypothermia are common in severe poisoning. Convulsions may occur, particularly in children. The presence of injection marks or venous tracking in an unconscious patient indicates that he is an addict and should arouse suspicion of opiate overdosage. Pulmonary oedema is a potentially lethal complication of mainlining narcotic analgesics and though relatively uncommon in clinical practice it is frequently found in those who die.

The speed with which features of narcotic poisoning develop clearly depends on the dose and the route by which it is taken, being faster after intravenous than after oral administration. However, concern has been expressed at the alarming rapidity with which dextropropoxyphene taken orally can produce severe coma, convulsions and fatal respiratory depression. Deaths have occurred within an hour of taking the overdose. It is not sufficiently appreciated that individuals taking preparations containing dextropropoxyphene may not survive long enough to reach medical care. This should be borne in mind when prescribing some popular analgesics to patients at risk of self-poisoning.

Treatment

Even if a narcotic antagonist is immediately available steps should be taken to ensure a patent airway and to support respiration if necessary. However, the need for endotracheal intubation and assisted ventilation can be obviated by the prompt administration of adequate doses of naloxone, a specific narcotic antagonist which has none of the partial agonist effects of nalorphine. It can therefore be given with complete safety regardless of the degree of certainty of the diagnosis of opiate poisoning. The optimum dose depends on the severity of poisoning and the drug taken and for an adult is usually at least 1.2 mg intravenously (0.4 mg for a child). Within 1–2 minutes or even less, the pupils dilate, the respiratory rate and minute volume rise, often transiently overshooting normal, and consciousness is regained. Hypotension is also reversed. The response is dramatic and it is not uncommon for intubated patients to sit up and extubate themselves.

Smaller doses of naloxone (e.g. 0.4 mg intravenously for an adult) are adequate for reversing the effects of therapeutic doses but are useless in the presence of a large narcotic overdose because they are insufficient to compete effectively at opiate receptor sites. The signs which indicate a positive response (pupillary dilatation and rise in respiratory rate) may then be minimal and missed, resulting in the patient being managed supportively.

Intubation and assisted ventilation are not without hazards and unnecessary exposure to even small risks is best avoided.

It should be noted that naloxone is the only narcotic antagonist which reverses the effects of pentazocine overdosage.

Failure to obtain a response to adequate doses of naloxone is an indication to review the diagnosis. However an absent or partial response may still be consistent with a diagnosis of opiate overdosage if the patient has taken other CNS depressants or has suffered hypoxic brain damage before treatment.

The effect of a single bolus of naloxone is short-lived and patients must be carefully observed for recurrence of coma and respiratory depression. Repeated doses of naloxone are almost always required and in some cases an intravenous infusion may be more appropriate. It cannot be emphasised too strongly that there is no fixed dosage schedule. The dose of naloxone must be titrated against the clinical response in each case and clinicians should not become faint-hearted if they have to exceed 'usual' doses. As much as 75 mg naloxone have been given in 24 hours without obvious adverse effects.

The indiscriminate use of naloxone as a therapeutic test for narcotic poisoning is not a substitute for intelligent appraisal of each poisoned patient. In Britain, a response to naloxone in a patient who is not obviously an addict raises the possibility of Distalgesic poisoning and is an indication to measure the plasma paracetamol concentration urgently. Patients who have taken enough Distalgesic to become unconscious from dextropropoxyphene have also taken sufficient paracetamol to be at risk of severe, but preventable, liver necrosis (p. 157).

Administration of naloxone to poisoned narcotic addicts may not only reverse the depressant effects of the drugs, but may also precipitate an acute withdrawal syndrome comprising abdominal cramps, nausea, diarrhoea, pilo-erection and vasoconstriction. While this is distressing, it is short-lived and seldom as severe as the mass media (and the patients) would have one believe and is obviously not a contraindication to the use of naloxone for the treatment of serious opiate poisoning in addicts.

Once patients have been resuscitated from the CNS depression caused by narcotic analgesics, the stomach should be emptied. The time limit for this procedure should be extended to 12 hours since opiates greatly delay gastric emptying.

References

Curtis JA, Goel KM. Lomotil poisoning in children. *Arch Dis Child* 1979; **54**: 222–225.

Ente G, Mehra MC. Neonatal withdrawal from propoxyphene hydrochloride. *NY State J Med* 1978; **78**: 2084–2085.

Hudson P, Barringer M, McBay AJ. Fatal poisoning with propoxyphene: report from 100 consecutive cases. *South Med J* 1977; **70**: 938–942.

Moore RA, Rumack BH, Conner CS, Peterson RG. Naloxone. Underdosage after narcotic poisoning. *Am J Dis Child* 1980; **134**: 156–158.

Young RJ, Lawson AAH. Distalgesic poisoning—cause for concern. *Br Med J* 1980; **280**: 1045–1047.

ORGANOPHOSPHATE AND CARBAMATE INSECTICIDES

Organophosphates

Azinphos methyl	Fenitrothion	Phorate
Carbophenothion	Fonofos	Phosalone
Chlorfenvinphos	Formothion	Phosphamidon
Chlorpyrifos	Heptenophos	Pirimiphos ethyl
Demephion	Iodofenphos	Pirimiphos methyl
Demeton-s-methyl	Malathion	Pyrazophos
Diazinon	Mephosfolan	Thiometon
Dichlorvos	Methidathion	Thionazin
Dichlofenothion	Mevinphos	Triazophos
Dimethoate	Omethoate	Trichlorphon
Disulfoton	Oxydemeton-methyl	Vamidothion
Ethion	Parathion	

Carbamates

Aldicarb	Methomyl	Propoxur
Carbaryl	Oxamyl	Thiofanox
Methiocarb	Pirimicarb	

General considerations

Organophosphate and carbamate insecticides are used extensively in agriculture and horticulture throughout the world and have caused human poisoning and death in many countries. Acute poisoning with these compounds occurs in a variety of ways. They are frequently taken deliberately, usually by ingestion although there are occasional reports of self-injection. Accidental poisoning is also common and outbreaks of poisoning have occurred when flour and other foodstuffs have been contaminated, particularly with organophosphates. Poisoning may also occur when these substances are being used for their proper purpose though the risk is negligible if the manufacturer's recommendations on preparation of solutions and safety precautions are heeded. Unfortunately, environmental factors, particularly high temperatures, encourage users to ignore wearing masks and protective clothing and risk poisoning by inhalation of spray or by percutaneous absorption. The latter usually results from failure to change soiled clothing immediately and from leaking spray equipment carried on the back as well as direct dermal contamination.

Organophosphates and carbamates act by inhibiting cholinesterases causing accumulation of acetylcholine at central and peripheral cholinergic nerve endings. Some are directly toxic while others (e.g. parathion and malathion) have to be metabolised before being effective. Carbamates produce relatively short-lived inhibition of cholinesterase since the carbamate-enzyme complex tends to dissociate spontaneously. In contrast, the duration of inhibition by organophosphates varies considerably from one member of the class to another but, in general, is much longer than with carbamates. The phosphorylated enzyme complex is comparatively stable and, with some organophosphates, 'ages' by a process of dealkylation. Recovery of cholinesterase activity then depends on synthesis of new enzyme by the liver which may take days or weeks.

Features

A garlic-like odour may be present from the poison. Skin exposed to organophosphate solutions for a few hours may become red and blistered. Accidental splashes in the eye will produce miosis and blurring of vision on the affected side.

Mild exposure may produce sub-clinical poisoning in which there is reduction of cholinesterase activity but no symptoms or signs.

The speed of onset of symptoms depends on the route and magnitude of exposure. Inhalation and ingestion may produce local bronchial and gastrointestinal effects respectively within minutes but systemic features take longer to develop. However they are usually apparent within a few hours if a large dose is involved. The onset of systemic toxicity is slowest by the percutaneous route.

The features of organophosphate and carbamate poisoning are a blend of peripheral muscarinic effects of excess acetylcholine on the gastrointestinal tract, bronchi, heart, bladder and sweat, salivary and lachrimal glands; nicotinic actions at neuromuscular junctions and sympathetic ganglia; and CNS effects.

Mild poisoning is characterised by CNS stimulant effects including anxiety, restlessness, insomnia, nightmares, tiredness, dizziness, headache and muscarinic features such as nausea, vomiting, abdominal colic, diarrhoea, tenesmus, sweating, hypersalivation and chest tightness. Miosis may be present.

In addition to these symptoms, the patient who is moderately poisoned shows nicotinic effects, particularly muscle fasciculation, and generalised weakness sufficient to make walking impossible and speech diffcult.

Consciousness is impaired in severe poisoning and there is widespread flaccid paresis of limb muscles (affecting proximal groups more than distal ones), respiratory muscles and (less commonly) various combinations of extraocular muscles. Patients who show severe muscle weakness early in the course of poisoning may have extensor plantar responses whereas those in whom paralytic features are delayed till about 24 hours after ingestion do not. The significance of this finding is not understood. Pulmonary oedema and cyanosis are common in severe poisoning and frothy secretions may pour from the mouth and nose embarrassing respiration further. Convulsions may occur. Complete heart block, atrial fibrillation and other unspecified dysrhythmias have been reported infrequently.

In the absence of a history of exposure the diagnosis of organophosphate and carbamate poisoning may be very difficult. The prominent gastrointestinal symptoms with fever and polymorph leukocytosis may lead to an erroneous diagnosis of gastroenteritis. Miosis is an important diagnostic sign but in 10 per cent or more of cases the diameter of the pupil is normal or even increased when nicotinic effects predominate. Similarly tachycardia and raised blood pressure are commoner than bradycardia and hypotension which occur late, if at all. Diagnosis may be further confused by the frequent finding of hyperglycaemia and glycosuria though ketonuria is absent.

Plasma cholinesterase activity

Measurement of plasma cholinesterase activity is useful for confirming a diagnosis of organophosphate or carbamate poisoning. In subclinical poisoning activity may be reduced by up to 50 per cent. Mild, moderate and severe acute poisoning are associated with reduction of cholinesterase activity to approximately 20–50 per cent, 10–20 per cent and < 10 per cent of normal respectively.

Treatment

The removal of soiled clothing and thorough washing of contaminated skin with soap and water prevents further absorption. The stomach should be emptied if the poison has been ingested.

Blood should be taken for estimation of cholinesterase activity in every case, preferably before starting treatment.

Treatment is unnecessary for subclinical poisoning but the patient should be kept under observation for about 12 hours to ensure that delayed toxicity does not develop.

Symptomatic poisoning is treated with atropine to antagonise the muscarinic effects of excess acetylcholine. It should be given intravenously in doses of 2 mg every 10–30 minutes depending on the severity of poisoning till signs of atropinisation (flushed dry skin, tachycardia, dilated pupils and dry mouth) are obvious. The total dose required in the first 24 hours is commonly as much as 30 mg and occasionally much more is necessary. Oximes such as pralidoxime (P2S, PAM, 2-PAM, P2AM) or obidoxime (Toxogonin) reactivate phosphorylated cholinesterase provided they are given within 12–24 hours but are contraindicated in carbamate poisoning.

Pralidoxime is given in a dose of 1 g by slow intravenous injection. Its effects will usually be apparent within 30 minutes and include disappearance of convulsions and fasciculation, improvement in muscle power and recovery of consciousness. The dose should be repeated after this time if satisfactory reversal has not been obtained. Further doses may be required at intervals thereafter but patients who relapse frequently may respond better to a continuous infusion of up to 0.5 g/h. The administration of pralidoxime usually necessitates reduction of the amount of atropine given and may unmask atropine toxicity. Pralidoxime has been used more extensively than obidoxime but they are probably of comparable efficacy.

It must be emphasised that the patient who is severely poisoned by organophosphates or carbamates requires energetic supportive measures in addition to atropine and oximes. Respiratory secretions must be effectively removed and endotracheal intubation may be necessary. Hypoxia must be corrected, particularly when large doses of atropine are being given. The adequacy of ventilation should be assessed by arterial blood gas analysis and assisted respiration started if necessary.

Fluids lost by vomiting, diarrhoea and in pulmonary oedema should be replaced.

Prognosis

Severe poisoning with organophosphates is usually fatal within 24 hours if untreated. Even with treatment a small proportion of cases die within days because of failure to respond significantly to adequate doses of atropine and pralidoxime. Complete recovery should follow treatment of moderate and mild poisoning. Long-term consequences of acute poisoning are uncommon but include peripheral neuropathy and less well defined symptoms such as tiredness, insomnia, inability to concentrate, depression and irritability.

References

Done AK. The toxic emergency: anticholinesterases. *Emerg Med* 1979; **11**: 167–175.

Gadoth N, Fisher A. Late onset of neuromuscular block in organophosphorus poisoning. *Ann Intern Med* 1978; **88**: 654–655.

Hayes MMM, Van der Westhuizen NG, Gelfand M. Organophosphate poisoning in Rhodesia. *S Afr Med J* 1978; **54**: 230–234.

PARACETAMOL (ACETAMINOPHEN)

General considerations

The toxicity of paracetamol in overdosage was first appreciated in 1966 when reports of jaundice and fatal hepatic necrosis were published. It soon became apparent that the liver damage was a dose-related effect. Paracetamol has been increasingly used for self-poisoning in Britain over the past decade and is presently involved in about 12 per cent of hospital admissions for this reason, being commoner than salicylate poisoning. This development is due to a combination of factors including substitution of paracetamol for aspirin because of concern about salicylate-induced gastritis and bleeding, the replacement of phenacetin by paracetamol in over-the-counter analgesics and the rapidly increasing availability of Distalgesic (paracetamol in combination with dextropropoxyphene), which in 1979 was the most commonly prescribed analgesic in Britain. Distalgesic now accounts for at least 40 per cent of overdoses involving paracetamol. Paracetamol (acetaminophen) poisoning has recently been recognised as an increasing problem in the United States and other countries.

The mechanism of paracetamol toxicity has now been elucidated. In therapeutic doses it is metabolised in the liver, largely to inactive sulphate and glucuronide conjugates. However, about 8 per cent is converted into a highly toxic intermediate metabolite which is normally immediately inactivated by conjugation with hepatic reduced glutathione and eventually excreted in the urine as cysteine and mercapturic acid conjugates. After overdosage, however, increased amounts of this metabolite are formed and rapidly deplete the limited hepatic stores of glutathione. It is then free to bind irreversibly with macromolecules in the hepatocytes producing necrosis. There is clinical and experimental evidence that drugs which induce hepatic microsomal oxidase (e.g. barbiturates and ethanol) increase susceptibility to paracetamol toxicity by increasing the rate of production of the toxic metabolite. Similar events take place in renal tubular cells. Children, however, seem less susceptible to paracetamol hepatotoxicity and this may reflect differences in metabolic pathways.

Features

The early clinical features of paracetamol poisoning are unremark-able. Nausea and vomiting are frequent within a few hours of the overdose and there may be generalised abdominal pain secondary to the effort of retching and liver tenderness. Loss of consciousness is not a feature unless Distalgesic or other CNS depressants have been taken. Patients frequently look paler and more miserable and have more protracted nausea and vomiting after reversal of coma in Distalgesic poisoning. These features are due to dextropropoxyphene rather than paracetamol and usually subside within 24 hours.

It is unusual for paracetamol hepatotoxicity to be clinically apparent before 12–36 hours. The usual warning signs comprise continuation of vomiting, localisation of abdominal pain to the right subcostal area and the presence of liver tenderness. Early renal tubular necrosis may also cause renal angle pain at this stage. Jaundice does not usually become obvious before the third or fourth day. If hepatocellular necrosis is extensive, hepatic failure ensues on about the fourth or fifth day (though occasionally sooner) with impaired consciousness, confusion, hyperventilation, hypogly-caemia and bleeding secondary to coagulation abnormalities. Fatal cases often develop respiratory or Gram-negative infections, cerebral oedema and disseminated intravascular coagulation. Acute renal failure occurs in a small proportion of patients, usually, but not always, those with severe liver damage and hepatic failure. Paracetamol causes renal tubular necrosis in the same way as it produces hepatic necrosis. In addition renal failure is common in hepatic encephalopathy from any cause.

The serum alanine and aspartate aminotransferase (ALT and AST) levels may begin to rise as early as 12 hours but peak values are not usually attained until 72–96 hours after the overdose. Aminotransferase activity of up to 10 000 units/l is common but elevation of the alkaline phosphatase is usually minimal. Plasma bilirubin concentrations rise more slowly than the enzymes and seldom exceed 190 μmol/l (10 mg/dl) in survivors. The prothrombin time ratio is often abnormal within 24–36 hours (maximum 48–72 hours). Hyperglycaemia is occasionally found in some jaundiced patients but with hepatic failure severe hypoglycaemia may occur. Plasma creatinine concentrations rise more rapidly than the urea when renal failure develops.

Haemolytic anaemia, methaemoglobinaemia, skin rashes, pancreatitis and myocardial necrosis have been reported in the literature as being features of paracetamol poisoning but they have not been encountered in the author's experience of many hundreds of cases. However, elevation of serum amylase levels has been documented and is to be expected since amylase is normally removed from the circulation by the liver.

Plasma paracetamol concentrations

The severity of paracetamol overdosage is best assessed from the plasma paracetamol concentration related to the time from ingestion. About 90 per cent of untreated patients whose plasma paracetamol concentrations related to time lie above line A (Fig. 4.1) develop ALT levels above 1000 units/l and most fatal cases and some of those who develop acute renal failure also come into this group. If all patients above line B are considered the proportion with plasma ALT above 1000 is about 60 per cent compared with only 25 per cent for those between lines B and C. In interpreting plasma paracetamol concentrations attention should be paid to the following:

1. Laboratory methods must be specific. Some colorimetric methods measure metabolites in addition to active drug, and may give values as much as seven times the actual concentration and thus mislead the clinician.

2. Plasma concentrations taken within 4 hours of ingestion cannot

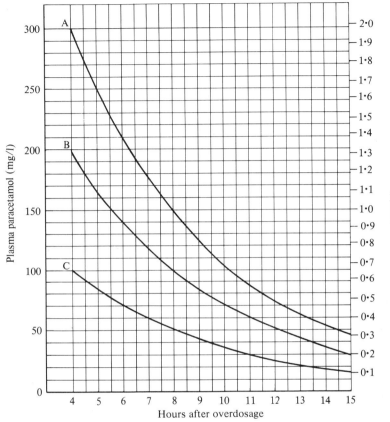

FIG. 4.1. Patients whose plasma paracetamol concentrations related to time from ingestion are above line B require specific treatment.

be reliably interpreted because the drug is still being absorbed and distributed.

3. The validity of line B beyond 15 hours is uncertain because of the paucity of data from untreated patients. However there is no doubt that patients who present late tend to be severely poisoned and at greater risk of serious liver damage.

4. It should not be assumed that the time–plasma paracetamol–liver damage relationship applies equally to Distalgesic poisoning since dextropropoxyphene is a narcotic and delays gastric emptying. Higher plasma concentrations are therefore obtained later than they would have been had paracetamol been taken alone. Patients who

have late high plasma concentrations after Distalgesic overdosage do not seem to develop liver damage as frequently as expected.

Treatment

It has been shown clinically and experimentally that paracetamol-induced liver damage, renal failure and death can be prevented by the administration of sulphydryl donors such as cysteamine, methionine and N-acetylcysteine although their mode of action is uncertain. Cysteamine (intravenously) was the first of these to be tried in clinical practice and though it was highly effective if given within 10 hours, it had distressing adverse effects and has been superseded by N-acetylcysteine. The latter provides virtually complete protection against liver damage when given to those at risk within 8 hours of the overdose but its efficacy declines thereafter. However, there is still considerable protection up to 10 hours and even from 10–12 hours but, like other sulphydryl donors, N-acetylcysteine seems completely ineffective if given later than 15 hours after ingestion. Intravenous N-acetylcysteine rarely cause any significant adverse effect and it should be regarded as the treatment of choice for severe paracetamol poisoning. Parenteral methionine is less effective.

Oral methionine is advocated in some centers (2.5 g 4 hourly to a total of 10 g, provided the first dose can be given within 10 hours of ingestion) but in one study 10 per cent of patients treated in this way subsequently had AST levels above 1000 units/l. Oral N-acetylcysteine has also been tried but the high incidence of vomiting in patients requiring treatment must necessarily raise doubts about the reliability of oral therapy.

The patient presenting with paracetamol poisoning within 15 hours of ingestion should be managed as follows:

1. Blood should be taken immediately (or at 4 hours after ingestion if the patient presents earlier than this) for urgent estimation of the plasma paracetamol concentration.

2. The stomach should be emptied while waiting for the laboratory result if more than 7.5 g have been taken within 4 hours.

3. The plasma paracetamol concentrations should be related to the time from ingestion and if the value lies above line B in Figure 4.1 intravenous N-acetylcysteine (Parvolex) should be started immediately. The dose is 150 mg/kg in 200 ml of 5% dextrose over

15 minutes followed by 50 mg/kg in 0.5 litre 5% dextrose over 4 hours and the same dose given over each of the subsequent two 8 hour periods.

4. If the patient presents at about the critical ingestion–treatment interval of 8 hours or at any interval from 8–15 hours after ingestion of > 7.5 g paracetamol N-acetylcysteine should be started immediately without waiting for the result of the plasma paracetamol concentration. If the latter subsequently suggests that the likelihood of liver damage is low, treatment can be stopped. This policy will inevitably result in the unnecessary treatment of some patients but is justified by the apparent lack of serious toxicity of N-acetylcysteine and the need to minimise hepatic damage (with a possibly fatal outcome) in those at risk.

Patients who present later than 15 hours after a paracetamol overdose should be managed supportively. There is no evidence that any sulphydryl donor can prevent liver damage at this late stage and they may contribute to the development of hepatic encephalopathy. Those at serious risk must have liver and renal function monitored daily. The single most useful investigation is the prothrombin time ratio (PTR) which should be measured daily together with standard biochemical tests of liver function until the expected time of peak liver damage is passed (i.e. the fourth day after ingestion). The PTR may have to be measured more frequently if it is rising rapidly or exceeds 3.0. In these cases fresh frozen plasma or clotting factor concentrates should be given to reduce the PTR and hopefully prevent haemorrhagic complications. Cimetidine may also be helpful and though vitamin K_1 can be given it is unlikely to be effective.

At the first indication of serious PTR prolongation (> 3.0) prophylaxis against hepatic encephalopathy must be started. This includes limiting the daily protein intake to 20 g, oral lactulose and neomycin to sterilise the gut and avoidance of CNS depressant drugs. The patient must be regularly screened for evidence of infection, hypoglycaemia and renal failure. The best guides to renal function are the urine output and plasma creatinine. The plasma urea may not rise until relatively late since urea production is diminished by extensive hepatic necrosis. Careful control of fluid and electrolyte balance is essential. Haemodialysis may be required for renal failure.

Prognosis

The mortality from paracetamol poisoning is very low but if deaths are to be avoided, doctors must be aware of the dangers of this drug, that an effective antidote is available and, above all, that treatment is a matter of great urgency. Patients who recover from paracetamol-induced hepatic necrosis regain normal liver histology without evidence of cirrhosis. Likewise, recovery of renal function should be complete. Patients with liver damage should be advised against consumption of alcohol for three months.

Reference

Prescott LF, Illingworth RN, Critchley JAJH, Stewart MJ, Adam RD, Proudfoot AT. Intravenous N-acetylcysteine: the treatment of choice for paracetamol poisoning. *Br Med J* 1979; **2**: 1097–1100.

PARAQUAT

General considerations

Paraquat is a bipyridilium herbicide which attracted much concern following a number of deaths from accidental ingestion of what appeared to be very small quantities of the 20% solution, Gramoxone, in the late 1960's. The high mortality, the publicity surrounding its subsequent use for homicide and the not unjustified belief that little could be done to influence the course of poisoning, added to its notoriety. Over the last few years, however, accidental paraquat poisoning in Britain has become uncommon and deliberate self-poisoning now accounts for most cases. Though paraquat poisoning is the mode of death for a substantial number of suicides throughout the world, proper use produces incalculable benefits by improving agricultural productivity in developing countries where it is used extensively. Some products and their contents are shown in Table 4.4.

Measurement of serial plasma paraquat concentrations in poisoned humans indicates that an uncertain proportion of paraquat is absorbed extremely rapidly from the gastrointestinal tract. Little is known of its distribution to tissues after absorption but there is experimental evidence of energy-dependent accumulation in some organs, particularly lung. Faecal excretion of paraquat continues for

TABLE 4.4   Liquid and granular products containing paraquat.

Product	Formulation	Paraquat ion content	Other constituents
Cleansweep	liquid	100 g/l	diquat
Cross Country Weed and Grass Killer	granules	25 g/kg	—
Dextrone X	liquid	200 g/l	—
Dexuron	liquid	100 g/l	—
Gramonol	liquid	100 g/l	monolinuron
Gramoxone	liquid	200 g/l	—
Gramoxone S	liquid	200 g/l	—
Herbex	granules	25 g/kg	diquat
Ortho Paraquat	liquid	2 lb/US gal	—
Pathclear	granules	25 g/kg	diquat, simazine
Sweep	liquid	250 g/l	—
Terraklene	liquid	100 g/l	simazine
Tota-Col	liquid	100 g/l	diuron
Total	granules	25 g/kg	—
Weed-ban	granules	25 g/kg	diquat
Weedol	granules	25 g/kg	diquat
Weedrite	granules	25 g/kg	diquat

several days in animals given one dose suggesting the possibility of entero-hepatic circulation of the poison. While some absorbed paraquat may be eliminated in the faeces, most is excreted in the urine, possibly by tubular secretion.

Sufficient paraquat can be absorbed percutaneously to cause serious and fatal systemic poisoning but this is very uncommon. In contrast, serious poisoning has not been reported after inhalation of sprayed solutions containing paraquat.

Solutions of paraquat are strongly alkaline and therefore corrosive but the mode of pulmonary toxicity after absorption is poorly understood. Paraquat is a multi-organ poison which has its most unique and lethal effects on the lungs, producing histological and functional changes similar to those of oxygen poisoning. Animal experiments have shown that the pulmonary toxicity is increased by high inspired oxygen tensions. This suggests that the toxicity of paraquat is due to the formation of superoxide radicals.

Features

The features of paraquat poisoning depend on the route and magnitude of exposure. A few exposure situations recur frequently.

Inhalation of spray of paraquat solutions often occurs in windy weather and when face masks are not being worn. Fortunately the consequences are seldom serious. A sore throat, husky voice and, in some cases, epistaxis, are usually all that develops.

Leakage from spray cannisters carried on the back has caused skin ulceration and a few patients have developed features of systemic poisoning (as detailed below). Five deaths have been reported from this type of accident.

Occasionally crops are eaten which have been recently contaminated with diluted paraquat. It is highly improbable that any individual could consume a sufficient quantity of the vegetable to be at risk provided the herbicide was correctly diluted before use. Should there be any doubt about the magnitude of exposure, urine and blood paraquat concentrations can be checked as below.

Potentially lethal poisoning occurs most commonly after deliberate ingestion of 1.5 g or more of paraquat, the amount contained in one sachet of Weedol or a small mouthful of Gramoxone. Paraquat has four major effects including corrosion of the gastrointestinal tract, hepatic necrosis, renal tubular necrosis and a complex sequence of pulmonary abnormalities culminating in progressive intra-alveolar fibrosis. The severity of these lesions and the speed with which each develops depends largely on the quantity of paraquat ingested. Three types of clinical course can be identified.

The most rapid course follows ingestion of 6 or more grams of paraquat. Nausea, vomiting, abdominal pain and diarrhoea occur within an hour or so and the patient becomes cold, clammy and hypotensive, partly due to fluid loss and partly the result of myocardial depression. A metabolic acidosis is frequently present, consciousness may be impaired and convulsions may occur. Within 12–24 hours there is increasing breathlessness and cyanosis due to acute chemical-induced pulmonary oedema. Death follows quickly before buccal ulceration and hepatic and renal necrosis become problems. At autopsy the lungs are found to be oedematous and haemorrhagic.

The second course is more protracted and follows ingestion of 3–6 grams of paraquat. The early signs of gastrointestinal irritation are present but shock does not develop. The alimentary features usually subside within 24 hours by which time pain in the mouth and throat becomes prominent making it difficult to swallow, speak or cough.

The mucous membranes of the lips, mouth and tongue become white in colour before desquamating patchily to leave painful red, raw surfaces after about 3 days. Perforation of the oesophagus with subsequent mediastinitis has been reported and some patients have vomited pieces of oesophageal and gastric mucosa. Others have been found to have the oesophageal lining coiled in the stomach at autopsy. Laboratory evidence of hepatocellular and renal tubular necrosis is usually obvious by about 72 hours but jaundice is seldom severe unless the patient has pre-existing liver disease. In contrast, renal damage is usually severe and may require treatment by haemodialysis. Breathlessness, tachypnoea, widespread crepitations and central cyanosis may be present by 5–7 days after ingestion and progress relentlessly until the patient dies from hypoxia a few days later. In such cases the lungs show alveolar oedema containing fibroblasts but haemorrhage tends to be less obvious than in patients dying earlier.

The slowest course may follow ingestion of 1.5–2.0 g paraquat (the contents of a sachet of Weedol). Nausea, vomiting and diarrhoea occur and renal tubular damage is usual but tends to be mild. Liver damage of any consequence is uncommon. Complaints of pain in the throat occur frequently but frank ulceration is unusual. Respiratory involvement may not be apparent till 10–21 days after ingestion. Breathlessness, basal crepitations and bilateral chest X-ray opacities are the earliest signs and progress till the patient dies as late as five or six weeks after taking the paraquat, by which time the local corrosive effects and hepatic and renal necrosis have resolved. The lungs are found to be excessively heavy and rubbery as is consistent with extensive intra- and inter-alveolar fibrosis shown histologically.

Respiratory damage due to paraquat is usually, but not invariably, irreversible and fatal.

Urine screening test for paraquat

Detection of paraquat in the urine is a simple matter particularly if the urine has been voided within a few hours of ingestion. 5 ml of urine is made alkaline by adding sufficient sodium bicarbonate to cover the point of a knife followed by a similar quantity of sodium dithionite. If paraquat is present a blue colour develops immediately, the depth of colour increasing with the concentration of paraquat. A pale green colour may be obtained with diquat or low concentrations of paraquat.

The absorption and initial renal excretion of paraquat is so rapid that failure to obtain a positive test on urine passed within 4 hours of alleged ingestion can be interpreted as indicating that no significant quantity of paraquat has been absorbed. This simple test is therefore of great value in accidental exposure, e.g. inhalation or ingestion of very small quantities.

Plasma paraquat concentrations

In serious paraquat poisoning the likely outcome can be predicted from the plasma paraquat concentration related to the time of ingestion. Patients with concentrations above the line in Figure 4.2 are very likely to die despite the best current therapeutic endeavours. Plasma concentrations taken within 4 hours of ingestion are difficult to interpret and there are insufficient data to be certain of the position of the line beyond 25 hours after ingestion. However, any patient whose plasma paraquat concentration exceeds 0.1 mg/l after 25 hours is unlikely to survive.

Paraquat concentrations can be measured by radioimmunoassay or by colorimetry and a result should be available within 45 minutes of the laboratory receiving the specimen.

High plasma concentrations can be crudely confirmed in the ward sideroom by applying the urine screening test to 2–3 ml of plasma. The darker the blue colour which develops, the higher the plasma concentration and the less likely that any useful treatment can be given. A faint blue colour is given with 2–4 mg/l.

Treatment

If the patient is first seen outside hospital the single most useful therapeutic measure is to give Fuller's earth (200 ml of a 30% aqueous solution) or bentonite (200 ml of a 7% suspension in water and glycerine) to bind paraquat remaining in the stomach and thereby prevent further absorption.

On arrival at hospital blood should be taken for urgent estimation of the plasma paraquat concentration. The stomach should then be emptied if the patient presents within 6 hours unless the urine test 3–6 hours after ingestion indicates negligible absorption. Gastric

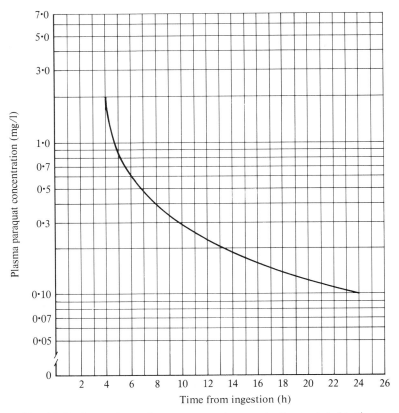

Fig 4.2. Patients whose plasma paraquat concentrations related to time from ingestion are above the line are likely to die, and those below survive. There are insufficient data to interpret concentrations measured within 4 hours.

aspiration and lavage is the method of choice since syrup of ipecac will be ineffective if an adsorbent has already been given. Fuller's earth or bentonite should be continued 2 hourly together with a cathartic to ensure rapid passage along the alimentary canal. Whole gut lavage has also been recommended but is time-consuming and frequently has to be abandoned because of persistent vomiting in the patients it might benefit most.

Anti-emetics and analgesics will be required in some cases and intravenous fluids may be necessary to replace gastrointestinal losses.

The plasma paraquat concentration related to the time from

ingestion should be used to guide further management. Patients whose levels fall below the line (Fig. 4.2) will almost certainly survive without additional treatment. Equally certainly, those with levels well above the line are extremely likely to die regardless of what is done for them. Forced diuresis and peritoneal dialysis are of no value and it is doubtful if haemodialysis or charcoal haemoperfusion can rapidly remove toxicologically significant quantities of paraquat. However they should be used in patients with plasma paraquat concentration close to the line in the hope that the elimination of even very small quantities of paraquat will tip the balance in favour of survival. To be most effective these procedures must be started as early as possible since plasma paraquat concentrations fall steeply during the first hours after ingestion. If there is any hope of influencing the outcome, dialysis should be continued intensively during the first 24–48 hours. The decision as to when to stop dialysis or haemoperfusion is difficult and should be guided by plasma paraquat measurements. The efficacy of these techniques will no doubt be assessed adequately in the next few years and their role in the treatment of paraquat poisoning may then vanish.

Corticosteroids, immunosuppressive drugs, and superoxide dismutase have also been tried but there is no evidence that they are of value.

Patients who are likely to die should be treated symptomatically and kept as comfortable as possible.

Prognosis

The mortality from ingestion of any quantity of Gramoxone is about 60 per cent and with Weedol (about a sachet or more) is about 10 per cent. Perhaps the most ominous feature is the onset of renal failure which effectively prevents the elimination of absorbed paraquat. Few patients survive paraquat lung damage. Since peak plasma concentrations of paraquat are usually achieved within a few hours, before most patients arrive at hospital, it seems that the outcome is already determined. Regrettably, current therapeutic measures are of doubtful value.

References

Proudfoot AT, Stewart MJ, Levitt T, Widdop B. Paraquat poisoning: significance of plasma paraquat concentrations. *Lancet* 1979; **2**: 330–332.

Rebello G, Mason J K. Pulmonary histological appearances in fatal paraquat poisoning. *Histopathology* 1978; **2**: 53–66.

Vaziri ND, Ness RL, Fairshter RD, Smith WR, Rosen SM. Nephrotoxicity of paraquat in man. *Arch Intern Med* 1979; **139**: 172–174.

PETROLEUM DISTILLATES AND TURPENTINE

Benzine	Mineral seal oil
Diesel fuel	Naphtha
Furniture polishes	Paraffin
Gasoline	Petrol
Kerosene	Turpentine
Lighter fluid	Turpentine substitute

General considerations

Petroleum distillates and turpentine are considered together because they have similar toxicological effects although they are chemically different. The term petroleum distillates refers to a group of solvents and fuels which contain differing proportions of a wide variety of aliphatic and aromatic hydrocarbons. Turpentine comprises a mixture of pinenes, camphenes and other terpenes and should not be confused with turpentine substitute (white spirit), a mixture of long-chain hydrocarbons which is extensively used as a paint thinner.

Ingestion of petroleum distillates is a common childhood problem because they are readily available in most households, including developing countries where kerosene, in particular, is used for heating, cooking and lighting. In both affluent and developing societies petroleum distillates are frequently kept in inappropriate, unlabelled containers thereby increasing the likelihood of accidental childhood poisoning.

Adults may deliberately ingest large quantities but are perhaps more likely to be poisoned accidentally in the course of siphoning petrol or gasoline from car fuel tanks. Petroleum distillates are also used as solvents for some pesticides and may add to their toxicity when ingested or inhaled.

Though ingestion is by far the commonest route for poisoning absorption of petroleum distillates by inhalation is also possible (see solvent sniffing, p. 201). Deliberate self-injection with these compounds has rarely been reported and systemic poisoning has followed the use of diesel fuel as a shampoo and for repeated hand washing.

Features

Ingestion of petroleum distillates usually produces remarkably little upset. Vomiting is common but no means invariable while diarrhoea is uncommon. Cerebral function is usually altered with some patients becoming excited and agitated but more often there is drowsiness leading to coma in severe poisoning. Convulsions occur rarely.

Most concern about petroelum distillate poisoning has centred on the pulmonary complications which occur in up to 60 per cent of cases and result from aspiration into the bronchial tree rather than from blood-borne hydrocarbon absorbed from the gastrointestinal tract. However, the higher blood concentrations attained by intravenous injection of these compounds may produce the same pulmonary changes as aspiration. The high incidence of respiratory complications in patients who do not vomit may be explained by the rapidity and ease with which some hydrocarbons with low surface tensions spread over large areas.

Clinical and radiological evidence of lung involvement is often apparent within minutes but in some cases may be delayed for up to 24 hours. Cough, choking, wheezing and breathlessness are the main symptoms and the smell of the hydrocarbon is usually detectable on the breath. Central cyanosis may be present but auscultation of the lungs is often unrewarding, even in patients with respiratory distress. Severe poisoning causes haemorrhagic pulmonary oedema which is fatal within 24 hours. Radiologically the pneumonitis usually involves two or more lobes and is occasionally perihilar in distribution.

Fever and a polymorph leukocytosis are common, even in the absence of a pneumonitis. Rare complications include pneumatocele formation, intravascular haemolysis and renal failure.

Diagnosis of hydrocarbon ingestion may be confirmed by finding a double gastric fluid level on an X-ray of the abdomen taken in the erect posture. This is produced by the layer of hydrocarbon floating between the gastric juice and the air bubble.

Treatment

The question of whether the stomach should be emptied after ingestion of petroleum distillates has been the centre of controversy for many years. While the tradonal assumption that induced vomiting and gastric lavage increase the incidence of hydrocarbon pneumonitis has been refuted by the majority of recent studies, there is equally no good evidence that they are of any benefit. Nevertheless, because of the risk of severe toxicity or the development of rare complications, present-day opinion favours emptying the stomach, provided the patient is sufficiently alert to be able to cough effectively or the airway can be protected by insertion of a cuffed endotracheal tube. The following are regarded as indications for gastric emptying:

1. Ingestion of > 1 ml/kg body weight (assuming a 'mouthful' in a 2 or 3 year old child to be of the order of 4–5 ml).
2. The solution contains another toxin (e.g. a pesticide).
3. Signs of serious poisoning are already present.

Administration of olive oil can reduce the absorption of petroleum distillates but unfortunately increases the incidence of pneumonitis and is not recommended.

Clinical and laboratory studies have failed to show any benefit from corticosteroids and routine antibiotics in patients with respiratory complications. Antibiotics should be reserved for those who develop proven secondary bacterial infection.

Oxygen may be necessary if cyanosis is present and intermittent positive pressure respiration should be considered for patients with pulmonary oedema.

Prognosis

The mortality from ingestion of petroleum distillates is considerably less than 1 per cent and death is invariably the result of hydrocarbon pneumonitis. The latter usually reaches its peak within 24 hours of onset and settles 3–4 days later. There are no reports of long-term lung damage.

References

Crisp AJ, Bhalla AK, Hoffbrand BI. Acute tubular necrosis after exposure to diesel oil. *Br Med J* 1979; **2**: 177.
Moriarty RW. Petroleum distillate poisonings. *Drug Ther* 1979; **9**: 135–139.
Neeld EM, Limacher MC. Chemical pneumonitis after the intravenous injection of hydrocarbon. *Radiology* 1978; **129**: 36.
Ng RCW. Using syrup of ipecac for ingestion of petroleum distillates. *Pediatr Ann* 1977; **6**: 708–710.

PHENCYCLIDINE

General considerations

Phencyclidine was originally developed as an intravenous anaesthetic for human use but was abandoned because of an unacceptably high incidence of postoperative psychotic reactions. It is comparatively easy to synthesise being considerably less expensive than other hallucinogens such as LSD. Phencyclidine has become a major drug of abuse in North America but has not yet been reported as a problem in the United Kingdom. It is often sold to unwitting buyers as THC or LSD. Although liquid and tablet formulations exist oral and intravenous use is uncommon. Phencyclidine is most commonly available as a white crystal-like powder which is smoked after mixing with tobacco or some variety of cannabis. Even among users it has a reputation for causing 'bad trips' and other side effects.

Features

The clinical features of phencyclidine intoxication are dose-related. If smoked it produces euphoria, perceptual distortions, numbness and parasthesiae, staggering and somewhat drunken behaviour. With higher doses, however, anxiety and agitation become prominent features together with hallucinations and muscle rigidity which makes walking slow and stiff. The pulse rate and systolic and diastolic blood pressures are commonly raised and hyperventilation and increased oro-pharyngeal secretions occur frequently. The individual may alternate between sitting rigidly with staring eyes and unpredictable violence. Deaths are most likely to occur during this phase of disturbed behaviour, drowning being particularly common. With increasing doses and particularly oral use, muscle twitching, facial grimacing, torticollis, convulsions and opisthotonus occur until coma, respiratory failure and paralysis supervene. Rhabdomyolysis has been reported after intravenous and oral administration. Tolerance and psychological dependence develop but an abstinence syndrome has not been described.

Discontinuation of phencyclidine may be followed by irritability, depression and impaired memory lasting several months.

Treatment

The stomach should be emptied if the drug has been ingested within the preceding 4 hours. Patients who are hyperexcitable should be stimulated as little as possible to minimise the risk of violent outbursts. Some, however, may require physical restraint till they can be adequately sedated. Haloperidol has been recommended but adequate doses of diazepam may be just as useful and also have the advantage of preventing convulsions. Severe tachycardia and hypertension may be controlled by propranolol. Unconscious patients require the usual supportive measures with particular attention to gentle removal of excessive secretions.

Urinary elimination of phencyclidine can be greatly increased by inducing an acid diuresis (p. 46). Disturbed behaviour can be expected during the recovery phase.

References

Barton CH, Sterling ML, Vaziri ND. Rhabdomyolysis and acute renal failure associated with phencyclidine intoxication. *Arch Intern Med* 1980; **140**: 568–569.

Corales RL, Maull KI, Becker DP. Phencyclidine abuse mimicking head injury. *JAMA* 1980; **243**: 2323–2324.

Crosley CJ, Binet EF. Cerebrovascular complications in phencyclidine intoxication. *J Pediatr* 1979; **94**: 316–318.

Sioris LJ, Krenzelok EP. Phencyclidine intoxication: a literature review. *Am J Hosp Pharm* 1978; **35**: 1362–1367.

PHENOBARBITONE

General considerations

While the incidence of barbiturate poisoning in general is declining, phenobarbitone overdosage is a continuing problem and will remain so in the foreseeable future because of its widespread use as an anticonvulsant. Indeed most patients who deliberately poison themselves with this drug are epileptics or close relatives of epileptics. Phenobarbitone poisoning is considered separate from poisoning by barbiturate hypnotics because its features and treatment differ sufficiently to warrant special mention.

Features

The dominant features of acute phenobarbitone intoxication are those of CNS depression but coma, if present, is seldom deeper than grade 2 or grade 3. It is unusual for patients poisoned with this drug to require endotracheal intubation or assisted ventilation and serious hypotension and hypothermia are uncommon. However the long plasma half-life of phenobarbitone (of the order of 3 days) makes recovery slow and symptoms persist for many days. Patients who are not unconscious remain drowsy, dysarthric and ataxic with gross, coarse nystagmus on the slightest movement of the eyes. Their management is made particularly difficult by their disinhibited mental state. They are frequently demanding, argumentative, loquacious, truculent and oblivous to reasoned discussion. They repeatedly insist on leaving when they are clearly very much under the influence of the drug and a potential danger to themselves and others. More than most patients recovering from drug overdosage, they are very likely to disrupt the normal functioning of medical units for several days.

Plasma phenobarbitone concentrations

Plasma phenobarbitone concentrations of up to 300–400 mg/l may be encountered in acute poisoning but they correlate poorly with clinical severity partly as a result of tolerance in patients (usually epileptics) already on long-term treatment. Plasma concentrations frequently continue to rise in the first 48 hours after ingestion during which time the patient may be improving clinically.

Consciousness with disinhibited behaviour is common with plasma phenobarbitone concentrations up to 100 mg/l or occasionally as high as 150 mg/l.

Treatment

Patients who are unconscious should be given supportive care.

If prolonged coma and other CNS effects are to be avoided it is essential to empty the stomach as thoroughly as possible in patients who have taken the tablets within four hours or in those who are unconscious.

The plasma phenobarbitone concentration should be measured as soon as possible though it is doubtful if there is much to be gained from requesting this as an emergency except in very severe poisoning when forced diuresis or other measures to increase elimination of the drug are being considered.

Forced alkaline diuresis is the treatment of choice for very drowsy patients and for those in coma.

A suitable regime for adults is 5% dextrose (0.5 litre), 0.9% saline (0.5 litre) and 1.26% sodium bicarbonate (0.5 litre) in rotation at a rate of 0.5 l/h. More or less bicarbonate should be given to keep urine pH (measured by narrow range indicator paper) in the range of 7–8. Bladder catheterisation is usually necessary to monitor fluid balance accurately and frusemide (20 mg intravenously) should be given if the urinary output falls more than two litres behind fluid input. Fluids should be infused at this rate until there is satisfactory clinical improvement (often two or three days). Apart from fluid overload, the main complications of forced alkaline diuresis are hypokalaemia and hypocalcaemia with possible tetany. The plasma electrolytes, including calcium, must therefore be measured at least twice daily and appropriate supplements given as necessary. It is also helpful to measure the plasma phenobarbitone concentration daily to ensure that the treatment is effective.

Patients in grade 4 coma, those in other grades who develop serious complications and those who are not responding satisfactorily to forced alkaline diuresis should be considered for treatment by haemodialysis or charcoal haemoperfusion provided the plasma drug concentrations are sufficiently high (p. 49). Charcoal haemoperfusion removes phenobarbitone more efficiently than haemodialysis.

The management of patients with behavioural disturbances due to phenobarbitone is difficult and may be dictated as much by the other responsibilities of the medical and nursing team at the time as by the needs of the poisoned patient himself. Sedation with chlorpromazine (50–100 mg intramuscularly) is usually effective and may be required while forced diuresis is undertaken to ensure rapid elimination of the phenobarbitone. However, the patient may not accept this and sedating him against his wishes raises difficult ethical problems. Such patients place a tremendous strain on the patience and good humour of the nursing staff who carry the brunt of placating and cajoling them into co-operating.

Prognosis

The vast majority of patients poisoned with phenobarbitone who reach hospital recover within a week with supportive care and forced alkaline diuresis. However, in severe poisoning coma may last several days and the risks of life-threatening respiratory infection are considerable, particularly if endotracheal intubation or assisted ventilation are required. Survival in these cases depends on energetic measures to remove drug rapidly from the body and good nursing care.

Reference

Bloomer HA. A critical evaluation of diuresis in the treatment of barbiturate intoxication. *J Lab Clin Med* 1966; **67**: 898–905.

PHENOTHIAZINES, THIOXANTHENES AND BUTYROPHENONES

Phenothiazines

Chlorpromazine	Perphenazine	Thiethylperazine
Fluphenazine	Prochlorperazine	Thioridazine
Mesoridazine	Promazine	Trifluperazine

Thioxanthenes
Chlorprothixene

Butyrophenones
Haloperidol

General considerations

Phenothiazines, thioxanthenes and butyrophenones have common pharmacological actions although the third group is chemically unrelated to the other two. Despite their widespread use for treatment of psychiatric illness, acute overdosage with these compounds is relatively uncommon. Chlorpromazine, thioridazine, trifluperazine or prochlorperazine are most frequently encountered. Occasionally self-poisoning with a combined preparation containing perphenazine and a tricyclic antidepressant is encountered and the toxicity of the antidepressant dominates although some features may be potentiated by the phenothiazine (e.g. cardiotoxicity).

Phenothiazines are perhaps more important in the context of self-poisoning because of the chronic disabling parkinsonian features which they cause in some schizophrenic patients. They are commonly being treated with injections of fluphenazine or fluphenthixol with or without oral phenothiazines. While the drugs may be controlling florid psychotic illness their adverse effects are occasionally so severe that they may be contributing to the difficulty the patient has in coping with life, whether or not anticholinergic drugs such as orphenadrine and benztrophin are also given.

Features

Overdosage with phenothiazines and related drugs causes CNS depression but profound coma and respiratory failure are uncommon. On the other hand they produce disproportionately severe hypotension and hypothermia. Some conscious patients show acute dystonic reactions including oculogyric crises, torticollis and orolingual dyskinesias, particularly with trifluoperazine, prochlorperazine and haloperidol. Other parkinsonian features are usually the result of long-term therapy rather than acute overdosage. Convulsions may occur.

A tachycardia is often present but conduction abnormalities and dysrhythmias are rare, although well documented, particularly with thioridazine. They may resemble those seen with tricyclic antidepressants. The PR, QRS and QT intervals may be prolonged and, rarely, bifid T waves are present. The most common reported dysrhythmias are ventricular tachycardia and fibrillation.

Death is usually due to cardiac effects.

Treatment

The stomach should be emptied if more than fifteen tablets have been ingested within the previous 4 hours. Treatment thereafter is symptomatic. Hypotension usually responds to elevation of the foot of the bed and intravascular volume expansion is seldom necessary. Cardiac dysrhythmias due to phenothiazines pose difficult therapeutic problems. Limited experience suggests that digoxin, phenytoin and lignocaine are of no value but these and other antidysrhythmic drugs may have to be tried in life-threatening situations. Attention should first be paid to hypoxia, acid-base disturbances and the plasma potassium concentration.

Dystonic reactions can be abolished rapidly by giving benztropine 2 mg or orphenadrine 20–40 mg intramuscularly or intravenously.

Forced diuresis, haemodialysis and haemoperfusion are of no value.

References

Donlon PT, Tupin JP. Successful suicides with thioridazine and mesoridazine. *Arch Gen Psychiatry* 1977; **34**: 955–957.

Lumpkin J, Watanabe AS, Rumack BH, Peterson RG. Phenothiazine-induced ventricular tachycardia following acute overdose. *JACEP* 1979; **8**: 476–478.

Scialli JVK, Thornton WE. Toxic reactions from a haloperidol overdose in two children. *JAMA* 1978; **239**: 48–49.

Sinaniotis CA, Spyrides P, Vlachos P, Papadotos C. Acute haloperidol poisoning in children. *J Pediatr* 1979; **93**: 1038–1039.

PHENOXYACETATE AND RELATED HERBICIDES

2,4 dichlorophenoxyacetic acid (2,4 D)
2,4,5 trichlorophenoxyacetic acid (2,4,5 T)
2 methyl 4 chlorophenoxyacetic acid (**MCPA**)
4 chloro 2 methyl phenoxyproprionic acid (mecoprop)

General considerations

Phenoxyacetate herbicides are used widely in agriculture for the control of broad-leaved weeds growing among cereals and are also available to the public for use in gardens. Though systemic effects can follow absorption through the bronchial tree, most instances of serious poisoning have been due to deliberate ingestion. Few cases have been reported but most were fatal.

Features

Initially there is burning in the mouth and throat followed by nausea and vomiting. The face may be flushed and there is often profuse sweating and fever. The most impressive effects are CNS depression with deep, prolonged coma, and hyperventilation which may lead to carpo-pedal spasm. Convulsions are uncommon. Fasciculation of the limb muscles and myotonia are usually present and on recovery the muscles are often painful, tender and weak. The latter may persist for some weeks after recovery and in the acute phase may involve the respiratory muscles causing ventilatory failure. Pulmonary oedema may develop.

A polymorph leukocytosis is frequently found and myoglobin and haemoglobin may be detected in the urine. The plasma urea may be elevated despite a good urinary output and muscle damage is reflected in raised serum levels of lactic dehydrogenase, creatine phosphokinase, aldolase and aspartate and alanine aminotransferases. Electromyographic changes consistent with a mild proximal myopathy were found in one survivor 6 days after ingestion.

ECG abnormalities have been reported.

Treatment

The stomach should be emptied and any necessary supportive measures instituted. The phenoxyacetate herbicides are moderately strong acids and forced alkaline diuresis considerably enhances elimination of 2,4D and, to a lesser extent, mecoprop. It should therefore be started as soon as possible if the patient is unconscious. The effect of forced diuresis on excretion of MCPA is not known. There are no published data on the efficacy of haemodialysis though one would expect these compounds to be freely dialysable. Since their volume of distribution is small, haemodialysis should be fairly effective.

Reference

Prescott LF, Park J, Darrien I. Treatment of severe 2,4-D and mecoprop intoxication with alkaline diuresis. *Br J Clin Pharmacol* 1979; 7:111–116.

PHENYLBUTAZONE

General considerations

Accidental and deliberate overdosage with phenylbutazone has been reported only rarely.

Features

Early features are due to CNS stimulation with agitation, irritability, jerking of the limbs and convulsions. Respiration may be rapid and deep and arterial blood gas analysis shows a respiratory alkalosis. Vomiting and epigastric pain are common. Drowsiness and coma may follow but these features usually disappear within 48–72 hours.

Oliguria, anuria and microscopic and gross haematuria due to acute tubular necrosis have been reported. Weight gain due to fluid retention was noted in one case.

Hepatocellular jaundice may become apparent 3–6 days after ingestion of the overdose but there are no reports of serious liver failure.

A polymorph leukocytosis is often present in the initial stages of poisoning.

Treatment

The stomach should be emptied if more than five tablets have been taken by a child, or ten tablets by an adult, within the preceding 4 hours. The blood urea, fluid balance and liver function tests should be monitored. Treatment thereafter is symptomatic.

Reference

Prescott LF, Critchley JAJH, Balali-Mood M. Phenylbutazone overdosage: abnormal metabolism associated with hepatic and renal damage. *Br Med J* 1980; **281**: 1106–1107.

PHENYTOIN

General considerations

Phenytoin (diphenylhydantoin) is widely used as an anticonvulsant and is commonly taken in deliberate overdosage by epileptics and their relatives and close friends.

Features

The features of phenytoin poisoning include nausea, vomiting, nystagmus, dysarthria, ataxia, drowsiness and, rarely, coma. Temporary abolition of the ocular responses to head rotation (the doll's head reflex) and ice-water stimulation of the ears at a time when the patients were able to carry out commands has been reported. The mechanism of this phenomenon is not understood.

Plasma phenytoin concentrations

Plasma phenytoin concentrations can be measured readily and values of up to 112 mg/l have been reported after acute overdosage. About 90 per cent of plasma phenytoin is protein-bound and at high concentrations the half-life is very long because of saturation of the drug metabolising enzymes. There is no merit in measuring plasma phenytoin concentrations as an emergency but daily measurement can be of value in estimating the duration of toxicity and timing the re-introduction of regular therapy in epileptics (the therapeutic range is 8–15 mg/l).

Treatment

There is no specific treatment for phenytoin intoxication. The stomach should be emptied if the overdose has been within 4 hours and supportive measures may be necessary if the patient is unconscious. Intravenous fluids should be given if nausea and vomiting are severe. Attempts to force a diuresis will not increase phenytoin excretion. Similarly peritoneal dialysis and haemodialysis are of no value.

Prognosis

The vast majority of patients poisoned with phenytoin survive although the plasma half-life of the drug is such that recovery may take several days. Occasional deaths have been reported and some investigators believe that permanent neurological damage can occur after a single acute exposure.

References

Rubinger D, Levy M, Roll D, Czaczkes JW. Inefficiency of haemodialysis in acute phenytoin intoxication. *Br J clin Pharmacol* 1979; **7**:405–7.

Wilson JT, Huff JG, Kilroy AW. Prolonged toxicity following acute phenytoin overdose in a child. *J Pediatr* 1979; **95**:135–8.

POINSETTIA

General considerations

Poinsettia (*Euphorbia pulcherrima*) is a house plant which is popular at Christmas because of its attractive red bracts and green foliage, which are commonly eaten by children. The milky sap of poinsettia is widely held to be toxic but there is little evidence to support this contention. Only fourteen patients in a series of 228 who ingested poinsettia developed symptoms. Although one child is reported to have died after eating leaves a recent review has cast doubt on the authenticity of the report.

Features

Little more than nausea, vomiting and diarrhoea are likely to develop after ingestion of poinsettia. On occasions these symptoms may be severe and dehydration may be a possible risk if the child is small.

Treatment

It is doubtful how energetic treatment should be. The stomach should be emptied if more than one or two leaves have been eaten. Most children will not require further treatment but symptomatic measures should be given if necessary.

Reference

Winek CL, Butala J, Shanor SP, Fochtman FW. Toxicology of poinsettia. *Clin Toxicol* 1978; **13**:27–48.

POTASSIUM CHLORIDE

General considerations

Acute overdosage with potassium chloride is surprisingly uncommon considering the vast quantities prescribed. However, deaths have been reported in children and adults after accidental and deliberate ingestion of large numbers of tablets, including 'slow-release' formulations. Dangerous hyperkalaemia has also followed the ingestion of salt substitutes. The principle toxic effect of potassium is on the myocardium and depends on the concentration gradient across the cell membrane and the rate at which it changes rather than the absolute plasma concentration. Thus patients who develop hyperkalaemia slowly are at less risk than those who attain similar levels acutely.

Features

Initially the patient may appear deceptively unaffected by an acute overdose of potassium chloride. Nausea and vomiting are common within a short time of ingestion but give no indication of the severity of poisoning. The most helpful investigations are the plasma potassium concentration and the electrocardiogram. The ECG manifestations of hyperkalaemia comprise peaking of the T waves, reduction of the amplitude of the P wave and PR prolongation till the P wave is lost in the preceding T. The QRS complex widens progressively and in severe poisoning may resemble a sine wave. Ventricular tachycardia may occur but death is usually due to asystole.

Treatment

The plasma potassium and urea must be measured urgently immediately on admission and at frequent intervals thereafter taking care not to haemolyse the samples. Arterial blood gas analysis should also be carried out to detect any metabolic acidosis.

The electrocardiogram must be monitored continuously. Evidence of cardiac toxicity requires immediate action and should take precedence over measures to prevent further absorption of potassium. Calcium gluconate (10–20 ml of a 10% solution) may be given intravenously to stabilise the myocardial cell membrane while the plasma potassium is being reduced and is indicated if there is QRS widening.

The potassium gradient across the cell membrane is reduced by shifting potassium from the extracellular fluid into the cell by giving dextrose (100 ml of a 50% solution) and soluble insulin (20 units) intravenously. Intravenous sodium bicarbonate (50 mmol or more) should be given to correct any metabolic acidosis and to produce an alkalaemia thereby facilitating the movement of potassium into cells. The extracellular potassium concentration can also be reduced by increasing elimination of potassium. The simplest way to do this is to force a diuresis by giving intravenous fluids and frusemide if the patient's cardiac state and renal function permit. If this is not possible urgent peritoneal or haemodialysis should be considered.

Once the patient's cardiac state has been stabilised the stomach should be emptied and an ion exchange resin such as calcium or sodium polystyrene sulphonate left in the stomach. They may also be given rectally.

Slow-release potassium preparations release potassium over 3–6 hours or even longer and in severe poisoning the use of whole gut lavage to eliminate tablets beyond reach of the stomach tube should be considered.

Reference

Illingworth RN, Proudfoot AT. Rapid poisoning with slow-release potassium. *Br Med J* 1980; **281**:485–486.

PRIMIDONE

General considerations

Primidone is an anticonvulsant which is toxic in its own right, apart from any contribution from its two active metabolites, phenobarbitone and phenylethylmalonamide. Acute primidone overdosage is uncommon.

Features

The features of primidone poisoning are those of CNS depression. Drowsiness, dysarthria, ataxia and coarse nystagmus are common and the patient may behave in a disinhibited manner. Rarely, coma, hypotonia, hyporeflexia, hypothermia, hypotension and respiratory depression may occur. A distinctive feature is the presence of whorls of shimmering white crystals in the urine. Surprisingly, renal failure has not been described.

Plasma primidone concentrations

Plasma primidone concentrations up to 100 mg/l have been reported after acute overdosage and decline with a half-life of about 15 hours. As the primidone concentration falls the plasma concentrations of phenobarbitone and phenylethylmalonamide frequently rise although the patient may be improving clinically.

Treatment

There is no specific treatment for primidone poisoning. The stomach should be emptied if more than fifteen tablets have been ingested within 4 hours. Supportive measures should be implemented if necessary. Elimination of phenobarbitone metabolite may be enhanced by forced alkaline diuresis although it has not been proved that this will hasten recovery from primidone overdosage.

References

Brillman J, Gallagher BB, Mattson RH. Acute primidone intoxication. *Arch Neurol* 1974; **30**:255–258.
Cate JC, Tenser R. Acute primidone overdosage with massive crystalluria. *Clin Toxicol* 1975; **8**:385–389.

QUINIDINE

General considerations

Quinidine is an optical isomer of quinine but its toxicological effects are sufficiently different to justify separate consideration. It is almost completely absorbed from the gastrointestinal tract and exerts its peak effects within 3 hours unless taken in a slow-release formulation. Poisoning may occur in the course of long-term treatment and as a result of deliberate self-poisoning.

Features

Nausea, vomiting and loss of consciousness may develop rapidly. Generalised convulsions occasionally occur and there may be respiratory failure due to a direct effect of the drug on the CNS. Intractable hypotension is common although the skin usually remains warm and dry because quinidine blocks peripheral alpha-adrenergic receptors.

The most serious effects are on the myocardium. Quinidine causes complex changes in ion transfer across the cell membrane, including a reduction of potassium efflux and increase in influx, the net effect being an increase in intracellular potassium and a variable degree of hypokalaemia. This results in potentially fatal changes in inherent automaticity, conduction, excitability and contractility. SA-block may occur but AV-block and intraventricular block are more common. The PR, QRS and QT intervals are prolonged. Cardiac rhythm may change frequently. A supraventricular tachycardia results from an anticholinergic action and, when combined with aberrant conduction, may be difficult to distinguish from ventricular tachycardia. Ventricular dysrhythmias, including ectopics, accelerated idioventricular rhythm, tachycardia and fibrillation have all been reported. Cardiac rhythm may change frequently over short periods of time.

Oliguria and a metabolic acidosis may result from hypotension and poor tissue perfusion.

Marked reduction of the plasma potassium concentration is uncommon but unexplained hypocalcaemia has been reported. A polymorph leukocytosis is frequently found.

Plasma quinidine concentrations

There is very little information on plasma quinidine concentrations after acute overdosage. It is often stated that cardiac toxicity is unlikely with concentrations of less than 8 mg/l. One girl survived coma, convulsions and cardia dysrhythmias with a peak serum quinidine concentration of 21.4 mg/l.

Treatment

The stomach should be emptied if any excessive number of tablets has been ingested within 4 hours. Arterial blood gas analysis should be carried out to ensure that ventilation is adequate prior to correcting any metabolic acidosis. Supportive measures may be necessary to protect the airway, improve gas exchange and control convulsions. Hypotension usually responds to cautious intravenous infusion of isoprenaline but if expansion of the intravascular volume is also required the central venous pressure should be monitored. An intra-aortic balloon pump was successfully used to maintain an adequate circulation in one case.

Potassium supplements should not be given unless hypokalaemia is severe (< 3.0 mmol/l) since hypokalaemia protects against the cardiac toxicity of quinidine. Ventricular tachydysrhythmias usually respond promptly to lignocaine or beta-blockers but cardio-depressant drugs should be avoided if at all possible. Cardiac pacing may not be successful because of a raised pacing threshold.

Techniques to enhance elimination of quinidine are of little value. The drug tends to be extensively bound in tissues. Up to 50 per cent of a therapeutic dose is excreted unchanged in the urine within 24 hours and this proportion may be increased by forcing an acid diuresis. Very limited information suggests that charcoal haemoperfusion may be beneficial. Although claims have been made for the value of haemodialysis and peritoneal dialysis the necessary laboratory confirmation is lacking.

References

Dellocchio T, Pailli F, Testa O, Vergassola R. Accidental quinidine poisoning in two children. *Pediatrics* 1976; **58**:288–290.

Shub C, Gau GT, Sidell PM, Brennan LA. The management of acute quinidine intoxication. *Chest* 1978; **73**:173–178.

QUININE

General considerations

Quinine sulphate is still widely prescribed for the prevention of nocturnal cramp and accidental and deliberate acute overdosage still occurs from time to time. Few cases are now due to attempts to induce abortion. Quinine is an alkaloid obtained from the bark of the cinchona tree which grows in some regions of South America. Cinchonism is the collective term for the common symptoms of quinine intoxication.

Features

The common features of quinine poisoning are nausea, vomiting, tinnitus and deafness. The skin is usually flushed, warm and moist. Visual impairment is probably the most dramatic feature and includes all degrees of severity from blurring to complete blindness developing over a few hours. The pupils dilate and become progressively less reactive to light as visual acuity decreases. The fundi are usually normal for the first day or two but by the third or fourth day after ingestion there is often retinal oedema, peripapillary oedema and attenuation of the retinal arterioles. Perimetry usually demonstrates severe constriction of the visual fields.

Some workers suggest that the visual abnormalities are the result of direct retinal toxicity while others maintain that they are secondary to quinine-induced arteriolar constriction and hypoxia. The latter view forms the rationale for the therapeutic use of stellate ganglion block (see below) and is supported by the dramatic improvement in vision obtained by some patients after this procedure.

Impairment of consciousness, convulsions and respiratory failure have been reported after ingestion of very large quantities of quinine. Similarly hypotension and cardiac dysrhythmias are uncommon, in striking contrast to their frequent occurrence in acute poisoning with quinidine, the *d* isomer of quinine.

Plasma quinine concentrations

Serum or plasma quinine concentrations of up to 8 mg/l have been reported after acute poisoning, usually in patients with severe visual impairment.

Treatment

The stomach should be emptied if the overdose has been taken within the preceding 4 hours.

Various measures have been used in attempts to improve impaired visual acuity but, not surprisingly, none has been adequately assessed clinically. Stellate ganglion block has been used most frequently and involves injection of local anaesthetic around the ganglion using a paratracheal approach at the level of the sixth cervical transverse process (about the level of the thyroid cartilage). This procedure is best carried out by an anaesthetist practised in regional block techniques and it is recommended that an interval of 30 minutes should be allowed before injecting the second side so that complications can be identified. These include haematoma formation, paralysis of the recurrent laryngeal nerve, intravascular injection, puncture of the dura and pneumothorax. The patients who have appeared to have the most dramatic visual improvement from stellate ganglion block are those who have immediately developed Horner's syndrome. The procedure may have to be repeated several times over a few days.

Little can be done to enhance the elimination of quinine since less than 5 per cent is excreted unchanged in the urine and it has a large volume of distribution. Forced acid diuresis has been advocated but it would not increase elimination significantly. Similarly, haemodialysis would not be expected to be effective. Fortunately quinine is metabolised rapidly.

Rare cases with coma, convulsions and cardiac dysrhythmias will require appropriate supportive care.

Prognosis

Death from quinine poisoning is rare and only likely to occur in patients with serious CNS or cardiac toxicity. Visual impairment is the only serious long-term complication and though improvement tends to occur, even without treatment, some constriction of the peripheral fields is likely to persist. Optic atrophy develops but permanent blindness has not been reported.

Reference

Valman HB, White DC. Stellate block for blindness in a child. *Br Med J* 1977; **1**:1065.

SALICYLATES

General considerations

Though salicylate poisoning has been a common clinical problem for decades, the mechanisms of many of its manifestations remain incompletely understood and it still presents diagnostic and therapeutic challenges. Accidental poisoning in childhood has recently declined in incidence following packaging of salicylates in child-resistant containers and deliberate self-poisoning in adults is showing a similar but less dramatic trend as aspirin is being superseded by paracetamol (acetaminophen) as the standard domestic analgesic. Unlike other drugs, about 50 per cent of the salicylate used for self-poisoning has been bought over-the-counter, often specially for the purpose. Fortunately methyl salicylate (oil of wintergreen) poisoning is now seldom encountered since it is several times more toxic than similar amounts of other salicylates.

Diagnosis of salicylate poisoning is usually straightforward but recent reports have drawn attention to difficulties when it complicates treatment of febrile illnesses in childhood. To some extent therapeutic intoxication results from the dose-dependent pharmacokinetics of salicyclic acid. Salicylates are well-absorbed and aspirin (acetylsalicylic acid) is rapidly hydrolysed to salicylic acid which is metabolised comparatively slowly to salicyluric acid and salicyl, acyl and phenolic glucuronides. The enzymes responsible are readily saturated within the range of therapeutic doses. Accumulation of salicylic acid is therefore very likely with large doses or frequent repetition of doses. The risk of therapeutic poisoning is increased if the hyperventilation, sweating, flushing and fever are erroneously attributed to the underlying illness and interpreted as an indication for further salicylate.

Salicylate poisoning may also occur by percutaneous absorption when salicylic acid ointment is applied extensively as a keratolytic agent.

Features

The clinical features of salicylate intoxication vary with age, young children tending to tolerate overdosage less well than older children and adults.

Salicylates commonly cause tinnitus, deafness, nausea and vomiting. Hyperventilation results from stimulation of the respiratory centre and salicylate-induced uncoupling of oxidative phosphorylation leads to increased oxygen uptake, carbon dioxide production and basal metabolic rate. Cardiac output is also increased with peripheral vasodilatation, bounding pulses and profuse sweating. Fever occurs in children but is seldom seen in adults. Some degree of dehydration is common.

Severe poisoning is distinguished by the presence of CNS features including delirium, extreme agitation, confusion, coma and convulsions. Impairment of consciousness is most commonly encountered in children below the age of two years and is rare in older children and adults. Indeed it is failure to lose consciousness together with the misery of salicylism which ultimately drives some adults to seek treatment after overdosage. CNS features in adult salicylate poisoning indicate a grave prognosis.

Complex acid–base disturbances develop and the resultant arterial hydrogen ion concentration is vital in determining the distribution of the drug. Since salicylates are weak acids, alkalaemia (reduced arterial hydrogen ion concentration) tends to keep the drug within the vascular compartment while acidaemia (raised hydrogen ion concentration) facilitates movement into the tissues, particularly the brain. Patients with CNS features are therefore usually acidaemic, although with very high plasma salicylate concentrations it is possible to develop the same features despite being alkalaemic. Reduction of the venous bicarbonate may indicate a metabolic acidosis but is more commonly the consequence of a respiratory alkalosis. Accurate assessment of the acid-base disturbance demands arterial blood gas analysis.

Arterial hydrogen ion concentration in salicylate poisoning depends on the balance of two opposing effects. Respiratory stimulation causes hyperventilation, reduction in Pa,CO_2 and a respiratory alkalosis; uncoupling of oxidative phosphorylation results in production of lactate and other organic acids of intermediary metabolism and a metabolic acidosis. Although both factors operate in most patients, children under the age of four years have a dominant metabolic component and often become acidaemic. In older children and adults the respiratory effect usually dominates and arterial hydrogen ion concentration remains normal or is reduced. In a small proportion of adults however acidaemia results and, as in young children, is commonly associated with impairment of consciousness.

It is traditionally held that the acid-base changes of salicylate poisoning occur in sequence, an initial respiratory alkalosis being followed by a metabolic acidosis. However in some cases acidaemia develops within 3 hours of acute poisoning and the respiratory alkalosis must be very brief or absent. The acid-base changes are not related to the magnitude of the plasma salicylate concentration.

Young women are particularly prone to develop subconjunctival haemorrhage and petechiae, usually on the eyelids, but occasionally more extensively over the face and neck. The precise cause of these is uncertain but they are probably due to a combination of reduced platelet stickiness and raised venous pressure associated with retching, vomiting and struggling during gastric lavage. They do not indicate a serious blood dyscrasia. Investigation is unnecessary and patient and relatives should merely be assured that the spots will fade in a few days. Despite the frequent occurrence of subconjunctival or dermal haemorrhage, retinal haemorrhages have not been reported. Significant prolongation of the prothrombin time does not occur.

Hypoglycaemia occasionally complicates salicylate poisoning in children but is very rare in adults. However animal studies have shown that brain glucose levels may be seriously reduced despite normal plasma concentrations although the relevance of this finding to human poisoning is unknown.

Rare complications of salicylate intoxication include gastric haemorrhage, tetany, non-cardiac pulmonary oedema, cerebral oedema, renal failure and oliguria, despite an adequate circulating blood volume suggesting inappropriate secretion of antidiuretic hormone.

Plasma salicylate concentrations

Plasma salicylate concentrations can be measured simply and rapidly. The features of salicylism are present at concentrations of 300 mg/l or more. Plasma concentrations of up to 800 mg/l are common and rarely values as high as 1700 mg/l are obtained after massive overdosage.

Plasma salicylate concentrations increase after admission in about 10 per cent of cases possibly due to absorption of drug flushed from the stomach into the small bowel during gastric lavage. It may therefore be necessary to measure the plasma salicylate concentration again a few hours after the initial estimation.

As indicated above, coma in adult salicylate overdosage is far from common and the indiscriminate measurement of plasma salicylate concentrations in all unconscious poisoned patients cannot be justified.

Treatment

The stomach should be emptied if more than fifteen tablets have been taken within four hours and the plasma salicylate concentration measured in patients with symptoms. Children with concentrations of less than 350 mg/l and adults below 450 mg/l do not usually require more than an increase in oral fluid intake. Patients with higher plasma concentrations but without CNS features should be treated by forced alkaline diuresis. A suitable regime for adults is 5% dextrose (1 litre), 0.9% saline (0.5 litre) and 1.26% sodium bicarbonate (0.5 litre) given in rotation at a rate of 2 l/h for 3 hours. Potassium chloride (40 mmol/h) should also be given to keep plasma potassium concentrations within the normal range. Frequently the onset of diuresis is delayed for 1–2 hours but this should not occasion undue alarm except in the elderly. Forced alkaline diuresis greatly increases the initial rate at which plasma salicylate concentrations decline although only relatively small amounts of salicylate are excreted in the urine. There is no doubt, however, that the symptoms of salicylism are more rapidly ameliorated by this treatment than by simply increasing oral fluid intake which may be impossible because of vomiting.

Acetazolamide has also been used to make the urine alkaline. It is undoubtedly effective and works rapidly but cannot be recommended because it also produces a systemic acidosis.

The management of very severe salicylate poisoning is more controversial. In many cases only a very limited amount of time (minutes or a few hours) is available for effective intervention since cardiac arrest may occur rapidly and without warning. Arterial blood gas analysis is mandatory and acidaemia should be corrected as a matter of urgency. Forced diuresis in such cases is likely to precipitate fatal pulmonary oedema and eliminates salicylate too slowly for such a critical situation. Haemodialysis rather than charcoal haemoperfusion is the method of choice for rapid removal of salicylate because it has the additional advantage of permitting removal of fluid if necessary.

If haemodialysis cannot be started immediately, curarisation and passive hyperventilation may have a temporary role in life-threatening salicylate poisoning. Hyperventilation, often gross, is invariably present and the work of breathing may be an important contributor to lactic acidosis and acidaemia.

It is also worth giving glucose (25 g intravenously) since animal studies have shown that brain glucose concentrations may be severely reduced despite normal plasma levels.

It is unnecessary to prescribe vitamin K routinely for salicylate poisoning.

References

Davies MG, Briffa DV, Greaves MW. Systemic toxicity from topically applied salicylic acid. *Br Med J* 1979; **1**:661.

Done AK. Aspirin overdose: incidence, diagnosis and management. *Pediatrics* 1978; **62**: Suppl 890–897.

Gabow PA, Anderson RJ, Potts DE, Schrier RW. Acid–base disturbances in the salicylate-intoxicated adult. *Arch Intern Med* 1978; **138**:1481–1484.

Heffner J, Starkey T, Anthony P. Salicylate-induced noncardiogenic pulmonary oedema. *West J Med* 1979; **130**: 263–266.

Temple AR. Pathophysiology of aspirin overdosage toxicity, with implications for management. *Pediatrics* 1978; **62**: Suppl 873–876.

SCOMBROTOXIC FISH POISONING

General considerations

Scombrotoxic fish poisoning is due to the accumulation of a heat-stable toxin in the flesh of red meat fish such as tuna, mackerel, bonito, skipjack and dolphin (mahimahi) which have been stored at insufficiently low temperatures. The spoiled fish usually contains excessively high concentrations of histamine which accumulate due to the action of bacterial decarboxylase on histidine. A variety of bacteria including species of proteus, *E. coli* and salmonellae have been incriminated. However scombrotoxic poisoning may occur in the absence of high fish histamine content and conversely when histamine concentrations are high poisoning does not necessarily develop.

Similar poisoning has occurred after ingestion of scombroid fish by patients taking isoniazid which inhibits histaminase.

Features

Symptoms usually start within 3 hours and often within a few minutes. Most can be explained by the action of histamine on smooth muscle and include flushing particularly over the face, trunk and arms, stuffy nose, burning of the mouth, throbbing headache, palpitations, pruritus, nausea, abdominal pain and diarrhoea. In severe cases breathlessness and wheeze may occur. Urticaria is uncommon.

Treatment

Treatment is seldom necessary and recovery is usually complete in twelve hours. Symptomatic treatment may be indicated in rare severe cases.

References

Cruickshank JG, Williams HR. Scombrotoxic fish poisoning. *Br Med J* 1978: **2**: 739–740.
Kim R. Flushing syndrome due to mahimahi (scombroid fish) poisoning. *Arch Dermatol* 1979; **115**:963–965.

SHELLFISH POISONING

General considerations

Paralytic or neurotoxic shellfish poisoning is uncommon. Sporadic cases and minor epidemics have been reported from various parts of the world including Alaska, Canada, West Europe and the United Kingdom. Poisoning usually follows ingestion of mussels and occasionally cockles or clams and is due to a water-soluble, heat-stable toxin known as saxitoxin. It is most likely to occur in spring and summer when a sudden increase in sea temperature leads to rapid multiplication of dinoflagellates, particularly *Gonyaulax tamarensis*, which discolour surface water leading to the description of waterbloom or red tides. These organisms are filtered by the molluscs which thereby concentrate the toxin.

Features

Symptoms may start within as short a period as 20 minutes or as long as 10 hours but generally within 3 or 4 hours. Circumoral parasthesiae and numbness are very common and may also occur in the fingers and toes and spread up the limbs. Frequently there is a feeling of dizziness, ataxia or floating and generalised muscle weakness may give rise to difficulty in moving and breathing. Vomiting and headache are less frequent features.

Treatment

There is no specific treatment for paralytic shellfish poisoning. Supportive measures are all that are required. The most important point is to ensure adequate respiration. Assisted ventilation may be required in severe cases. Complete recovery may be expected if the patient survives 24 hours.

References

Acres J, Gray J. Paralytic shellfish poisoning. *Can Med Assoc J* 1978; **119**: 1195–1197.
Ayres PA. Mussel poisoning in Britain with special reference to paralytic shellfish poisoning. *Environ Health Perspect* 1975; **83**: 261–265.

SMOKE

General considerations

People who are involved in fires are at serious risk even if they escape skin burns and thermal injury to the upper respiratory tract. Asphyxia is a hazard if the fire uses the available oxygen. Smoke is another potentially lethal cause of injury since it contains particles and toxic gases which, unlike heat, readily reach the alveoli. The gases present at fires vary considerably according to the materials involved and the temperature of combustion. Hydrogen chloride (from polyvinyl wall, floor and furnishing coverings), isocyanates (from polyurethane foams), acrylonitriles, phosgene, acrolein and a variety of aldehydes may cause alveolar damage and impair gas exchange while carbon monoxide reduces the oxygen-carrying capacity of the blood without causing chemical pulmonary damage and hydrogen cyanide prevents cellular oxygen utilisation. The role of inhaled particles (mainly soot) in the pathogenesis of pulmonary lesions has not yet been elucidated but may be unimportant.

Many patients will have pre-existing chronic obstructive airways disease from cigarette smoking. Many fires arise through smoking in bed, occasionally while under the influence of alcohol or drugs.

Features

Most patients who present to physicians will have minimal or no burns. Those with even minimal facial burns, singeing of the hair, eyebrows and eyelashes must be observed very carefully since they are at risk of thermal injury to the upper respiratory tract and may develop delayed severe respiratory obstruction due either to laryngeal oedema or expectoration of large sheets of desquamated mucosa. Damage does not occur beyond the main bronchi because air temperature drops very rapidly after inhalation.

Many patients will be covered in soot and smell strongly of smoke. Depending on the acridity of the smoke the eyes may sting and stream and there may be a metallic taste in the mouth. The voice may be hoarse and the throat sore and inflamed. Cough, wheeze, breathlessness and chest tightness are common complaints. The sputum often contains large amounts of soot. Rhonchi and crepitations may be heard on auscultation. Central cyanosis may be obvious. Many patients will have significant concentrations of carboxyhaemoglobin in their blood without the skin showing the 'typical' cherry red colour.

Arterial blood gas analysis immediately on arrival at hospital often reveals much more marked hypoxia than would be suspected from the symptoms and signs, unless oxygen has been given en route from the fire. Pa,co_2 is usually slightly reduced, reflecting hyperventilation, and the hydrogen ion concentration may be reduced or increased depending on whether hypoxia has been of sufficient severity and duration to produce a metabolic acidosis.

Carboxyhaemoglobin concentrations between 10 and 50 per cent are common but higher values are usually found only in fatal cases. The concentration on arrival at hospital may underestimate the severity of exposure since carboxyhaemoglobin will tend to dissociate as soon as exposure to carbon monoxide ceases, especially if oxygen is given. Plasma concentrations of cyanide and other toxins absorbed by inhalation during fires have seldom been measured.

The majority of smoke inhalation victims have normal chest X-rays but some have focal pulmonary infiltrates which clear in about three days, diffuse patchy opacities (which tend to resolve more slowly) or changes in keeping with pulmonary oedema.

The radiographic appearances correlate poorly with the degree of hypoxia and carboxyhaemoglobin concentrations which are better guides to the severity of smoke inhalation.

The electrocardiogram may show tachycardia and ischaemic changes.

Treatment

Reversal of toxic effects starts the moment the victim is removed from the smoke. Lives may be saved at the scene of the fire by simple measures to establish a patent airway and assist ventilation before transfer to hospital. High concentrations of oxygen in the inspired air should be given in the ambulance. These measures should be continued till the adequacy of ventilation and severity of exposure has been assessed by arterial blood gas analysis and measurement of the carboxyhaemoglobin level.

High dose corticosteroids have been recommended for a few days to minimise the chemical pneumonitis but their value is unproven. Steroids are indicated if cerebral oedema is suspected. In elderly patients and those with high carboxyhaemoglobin concentrations the ECG and plasma aspartate aminotransferase activity should be monitored to detect serious ischaemia or infarction.

References

Genovesi MG, Tashkin DP, Chopra S, Morgan M, McElroy C. Transient hypoxemia in firemen following inhalation of smoke. *Chest* 1977; **71**:441–444.

Oliver SA, Jaeger RW, deCastro FJ. Smoke inhalation: a poison center protocol for management. *Vet Hum Toxicol* 1980; **22**:84–86.

Putman CE, Loke J, Matthay RA, Ravin CE. Radiographic manifestations of acute smoke inhalation. *AJR* 1977; **129**:865–870.

SOAPS, HOUSEHOLD DETERGENTS AND FABRIC CONDITIONERS

General considerations

Soaps, household detergents and fabric conditioners are commonly ingested by toddlers. Soaps comprise sodium and potassium salts of fatty acids obtained from edible fats. Synthetic detergents are complex formulations of a variety of chemicals including surface acting agents (usually anionic or non-ionic varieties), mild alkalis (sodium silicate or sodium triphosphate) which comprise the bulk of washing powders, and bleaches (sodium hypochlorite or sodium perborate) in addition to perfumes, proteolytic enzymes, whiteners, stabilisers etc. The relative amounts vary according to the nature of the material to be cleaned and the conditions under which it is to be used (e.g. temperature, degree of mechanical agitation, etc.). The principal ingredient of fabric conditioners (intended to make clothes soft and fluffy) is a cationic detergent, often di-alkyl, di-methyl ammonium chloride. Fortunately the complexities of detergent formulations are clinically relatively unimportant.

Features

Only a minority of children who ingest these products develop symptoms. Except in rare cases where aspiration into the lungs occurs, features of ingestion are confined to the alimentary tract. Nausea, vomiting and diarrhoea are common but abdominal pain, haematemesis or rectal bleeding seldom occur. There may be discomfort or pain in the mouth but ulceration of the mucosa is unusual, even when the most alkaline of these products (automatic dishwashing detergents) are swallowed.

Treatment

There is no specific treatment for ingestion of soaps and detergents. It is unnecessary to empty the stomach. A good fluid intake should be ensured and demulcents such as milk may be helpful. It is seldom necessary to refer children to hospital after ingestion of these products.

Prognosis

Symptoms almost always disappear well within 24 hours.

References

Goulding R, Ashforth GK, Jenkins H. Household products and poisoning. *Br Med J* 1978; **1**: 286–287.
Temple AR, Veltri JC. Outcome of accidental ingestions of soaps, detergents and related household products. *Vet Hum Toxicol* 1979; **21**: Suppl 31–32.

SOLVENT INHALATION

Acetone	Methyl-ethyl-ketone
Butane	Methylene chloride
Carbon tetrachloride	Petrol
Chloroform	Tetrachlorethylene
Ether	Toluene
Fluorinated hydrocarbons	Trichloroethane
n-Hexane	Trichloroethylene
Lighter fluid (paraffin hydrocarbons)	

General considerations

The deliberate inhalation of volatile organic solvents for pleasurable effects (solvent abuse, solvent sniffing or glue sniffing) is most commonly found among young male teenagers. It is often a group activity. Many, but by no means all, have a background of emotional instability and come from broken or disturbed homes. Their academic performance is often poor and truancy is common.

Compounds such as those listed above are highly lipid soluble and therefore have marked effects on nervous tissue. They are available, singly or in combination, in a wide variety of household products including shoe cleaners, polishes, adhesive cements, spot and nail polish removers, dry cleaning agents, paint thinners, hair lacquers and antifreeze preparations. The substance is usually applied to a piece of cloth and held near the nose or emptied into a plastic bag, the opening of which is then gathered together and held over the nose and mouth. Solvents may be inhaled in this manner intermittently for several hours. Elimination from the body is mainly through the respiratory system but some solvents are metabolised, mainly in the liver.

Features

Solvents are inhaled for the CNS excitation ('buzz') they produce before causing depression. In the early stages they induce a sense of well-being and exhilaration which may include auditory and visual hallucinations. Dizziness and ataxia are common and there may be sneezing and coughing due to mild irritation of the respiratory mucosa. Behaviour may become abnormal and is dependent partly on the previous personality of the individual and partly on the reaction and activities of the group as a whole.

Increasing exposure causes progressive depression of consciousness with mental confusion, loss of self-control, ataxia, dysarthria and nystagmus leading to coma and occasionally convulsions. Severe hypoxia may develop and halogenated hydrocarbons sensitise the heart to endogenous catecholamines, and may thus cause fatal cardiac dysrhythmias. A severe metabolic acidosis may occur.

Sniffers are unlikely to come to medical attention while acutely intoxicated unless they are caught in the act, are creating a disturbance or develop some serious acute complication such as deep coma. However they may present later with other features which result from particularly heavy or repeated exposure. These include jaundice and renal damage (toluene, carbon tetrachloride and other halogenated hydrocarbons), acute and chronic encephalopathy (petrol with its tetraethyl lead content), cerebellar degeneration (toluene), or a predominantly motor, mixed polyneuropathy (hexane). The incidence of these complications cannot be determined with any certainty but is probably very small.

Treatment

Stopping solvent inhalation is all the 'treatment' most sniffers require for acute intoxication. As a result most have improved considerably by the time they reach hospital but some may require sedation if in a state of panic or if still excited or rowdy. Unconscious patients require supportive measures to ensure a clear airway and adequate ventilation and oxygenation. They should also have arterial blood gas analysis carried out and any metabolic acidosis corrected.

Hepatocellular and renal damage should be assessed biochemically and treated conventionally.

Prognosis

The prognosis for uncomplicated acute intoxication is excellent and complete recovery can be expected within a few hours of stopping solvent exposure. Renal and hepatic damage is reversible but long-term neurological complications are unlikely to improve significantly. Abstinence from further solvent abuse is vitally important.

References

Fischman CM, Oster JR. Toxic effects of toluene. *JAMA* 1979; **241**:1713–1715.

Horne MK, Waterman MR, Simon LaVM, Garriott JC, Foerster EH. Methemoglobinemia from sniffing butyl nitrite. *Ann Intern Med* 1979; **91**:417–418.

Watson JM. Morbidity and mortality statistics on solvent abuse. *Med Sci Law* 1979; **19**:246–252.

Watson JM. Solvent abuse by children and young adults: a review. *Br J Addict* 1980; **75**:27–36.

Valpey R, Sumi SM. Copass MK, Goble GJ. Acute and chronic progressive encephalopathy due to gasoline sniffing. *Neurology (Minneap)* 1978; **28**:507–510.

THEOPHYLLINE AND OTHER BRONCHO-DILATORS

Aminophylline	Salbutamol
Choline theophyllinate	Terbutaline
Ephedrine	Theophylline

General considerations

Deliberate self-poisoning with bronchodilators probably occurs more often than the literature would suggest and therapeutic overdosage is also common. In addition, some patients with respiratory diseases become dependent on the CNS stimulant effects of bronchodilators and take them orally or by inhalation to gross excess.

Some older, but still popular, bronchodilator formulations combine ephedrine (an α- and β-adrenergic agonist which occurs naturally in a wide variety of plants) with a xanthine derivative (theophylline or aminophylline) and a barbiturate. The latter is presumably intended to counteract the increased toxicity from combining the other two drugs—a combination which has no therapeutic advantage. The consequences of acute overdosage with these compounds are correspondingly complicated.

Salbutamol and terbutaline are selective β_2-adrenergic stimulants which are being increasingly used for the treatment of asthma, bronchitis and chronic obstructive airways disease.

Features

The xanthine derivatives cause marked gastrointestinal irritation with nausea, vomiting and occasionally diarrhoea. Haematemesis is also common and may be severe. Ephedrine, salbutamol and terbutaline are much less likely to produce these effects.

All bronchodilators cause CNS stimulation. The patient becomes restless, hyperactive and talks rapidly. Dilatation of the pupils is common and myoclonus, erratic jerky movements of the limbs, increased muscle tone and exaggerated reflexes usually precede convulsions which may be generalised or focal. Hyperventilation is an integral part of the increase in arousal. The generalised increase in muscular activity and brain stimulation commonly causes hyperpyrexia. These features dominate even when the preparation ingested includes a barbiturate, although the latter may produce coma at an early stage. Impairment of consciousness may eventually occur even in the absence of a barbiturate.

A tachycardia is invariable, even in mild poisoning. The blood pressure may be slightly raised in the initial phase but falls later if the heart rate rises considerably. Supraventricular and ventricular ectopic beats presage more serious tachydysrhythmias, including ventricular fibrillation. It is uncertain to what extent the cardiac effects are due to the drugs themselves or to the increased endogenous catecholamine secretion they cause.

A number of complex, inter-related metabolic disturbances accompany overdosage with xanthines and ephedrine. In the initial phases hyperventilation leads to a respiratory alkalosis but a metabolic acidosis develops as poisoning becomes more severe. Hyperglycaemia and glycosuria result from increased secretion of catecholamines which, together with theophylline, also stimulate lipolysis with subsequent elevation of plasma free fatty acid concentrations. Production of c-AMP is stimulated by ephedrine and its breakdown reduced by theophylline which is a phosphodiesterase inhibitor. These drugs therefore potentiate the effects of endogenous catecholamines causing hyperinsulinaemia and severe hypokalaemia as potassium is driven into cells. Salbutamol given intravenously in therapeutic doses has been shown to produce similar effects.

Plasma concentrations of theophylline and ephedrine

Plasma concentrations of theophylline and ephedrine can be

measured by high performance liquid chromatography and with therapeutic doses are usually of the order of 10–20 mg/l and up to 0.8 mg/l respectively. Theophylline concentrations up to 270 mg/l and ephedrine concentrations of 13 mg/l have been reported after massive overdosage. The plasma half-life of theophylline in such cases is about 9 hours.

Treatment

The stomach should be emptied if the patient presents within 4 hours of the overdose. The cardiac rhythm should be monitored continuously and appropriate supportive measures may be necessary especially if the formulation ingested contains a barbiturate and consciousness is impaired. A combination of coma, convulsions and vomiting is particularly hazardous. In such situations it is advisable to paralyse, intubate and ventilate the patient rather than give parenteral anticonvulsants. Assisted ventilation also allows rapid correction of hyperventilation and respiratory alkalosis which contributes to the intracellular movement of potassium. For similar reasons it is important not to over-correct any metabolic acidosis.

If the increased potassium gradient across cell membranes is important in the genesis of cardiac dysrhythmias it seems reasonable to correct marked hypokalaemia (<2.8 mmol/l) by infusing potassium chloride and correcting respiratory alkalosis, when present. Marked supraventricular tachycardia should be controlled with β-adrenergic blockers. Large amounts may be required to produce adequate competition for receptor sites and the dose must be titrated against the clinical response. Ventricular dysrhythmias are treated similarly.

It is important to keep in mind the possibility of gastrointestinal blood loss as a cause of hypotension and tachycardia. Monitoring of the central venous pressure and blood transfusion may be necessary.

The plasma half-life of theophylline can be considerably shortened by charcoal or resin haemoperfusion and the use of one of these techniques should be considered in suitable cases (p. 47).

Prognosis

Severe poisoning with theophylline and its derivatives carries a high mortality. Most patients who die have plasma theophylline concentrations above 65 mg/l. Convulsions indicate a poor prognosis.

References

Adam RD, Robertson C, Jarvie DR, Stewart MJ, Proudfoot AT. Clinical and metabolic features of overdosage with Amesec. *Scot Med J* 1979; **24**:246–249.

Helliwell M, Berry D. Theophylline poisoning in adults. *Brit Med J* 1979; **2**:1114.

Jefferys DB, Raper SM, Helliwell M, Berry DJ, Crome P. Haemoperfusion for theophylline overdose. *Brit Med J* 1980; **280**:1167.

THYROXINE AND TRIIODOTHYRONINE

General considerations

In 1955 an American review of accidental poisoning in childhood listed thyroid extract as the third most common drug involved. Today, acute overdosage with thyroid hormones is seldom reported, probably because it rarely causes serious effects. Most episodes involve thyroxine (T4) but recently acute overdosage with triiodothyronine (T3) has been reported.

Features

It seems likely that only a minority of patients develop significant toxicity after acute overdosage with thyroid hormones. Symptoms develop within a few hours with T3 but take 3–6 days following overdosage with thyroxine. One child developed toxic features within 6 hours of taking thyroid extract and in this case the rapid onset was presumably due to the T3 content. However, a woman who also took thyroid extract did not become ill for some days.

The principal effects are on the CNS and heart. Mental confusion, agitation, irritability and hyperactivity are common with mydriasis, tachycardia, tachypnoea and pyrexia. Other features of thyrotoxicosis, including atrial fibrillation, sweating, loose stools, lid retraction and prominence of the eyes appear to be uncommon. In most cases toxic features abate in the same time they took to develop.

The relatively benign and short-lived course of T3 overdosage probably reflects its much shorter plasma half-life.

Thyroid function test abnormalities

Serum concentrations of hormones depend on the dose ingested and the time since ingestion and may be many times physiological values.

TSH concentrations and I^{131} uptake are depressed within a few days but return to normal within two weeks.

A normal serum T4 more than 6 hours after ingestion precludes the possibility of delayed toxicity.

Treatment

The stomach should be emptied if more than fifteen tablets have been ingested within 4 hours. Blood should be taken 6–12 hours after ingestion for estimation of T4 and T3 concentrations. Patients with normal results may be discharged without follow-up. Those seen early and found to have high T4 concentrations should be reviewed for evidence of toxicity on the fourth or fifth day post-ingestion.

Propranolol will rapidly control all the features of overdosage. 40 mg orally 6-hourly may be sufficient but this may have to be increased depending on the response in individual cases. Treatment should only be necessary for 5–6 days after the onset of toxic features.

Plasmapheresis has been used to enhance the elimination of thyroxine after overdosage but seems unnecessary and extravagant when β-adrenergic blocking drugs are so effective.

References

Dahlberg PA, Karlsson FA, Wide L. Triiodothyronine intoxication. *Lancet* 1979; **2**:700.

Nyström E, Lindstedt G, Lundberg PA. Minor signs and symptoms of toxicity in a young woman in spite of massive thyroxine ingestion. *Acta Med Scand* 1980; **207**:135–136.

TOILETRIES AND COSMETICS

General considerations

Toiletries and cosmetics are readily accessible in most homes and it is hardly surprising that they should be commonly involved in childhood poisoning when children mimic their seniors. Toilet articles frequently contain several different potentially toxic compounds in relatively low concentrations. The usual principal constituents of the most common are listed in Table 4.5. Many are innocuous but others such as perfumes, colognes, after-shave lotions, mouth washes, hair removers, nail varnish and nail varnish removers

TABLE 4.5   The usual principal constituents of common toilet preparations and cosmetics.

Preparations	Constituents
*Skin preparations**	
After-shave lotion	Ethanol
Colognes	Ethanol
Deodorants	Aluminium or zinc salts
Eye and face make-up	Numerous, non-toxic
Hand cream	Lanolin
Lipstick	Waxes, oils, dyes
Perfumes	Ethanol
Shaving cream	Salts of fatty acids
Hair preparations	
Hair lacquer	Ethanol
Hair remover	Potassium thioglycollate
Shampoo (liquid)	Lanolin, Lauric diethanolamine, triethanolamine lauryl sulphate
Nail preparations	
Nail varnish	Toluene, ethanol, isopropanol, ethyl acetate
Nail varnish remover	Acetone, ethyl acetate, isopropanol
Bath preparations	
Bath crystals and cubes	Sodium carbonate and phosphate
Bubble bath solutions	Sodium lauryl ether sulphate

* Soaps are considered on p. 199.

are potentially toxic. The risk of consuming dangerous quantities, however, is reduced by presenting them in relatively small volumes.

Features

In general, ingestion of toiletries and cosmetics produces very few symptoms. Liquid shampoos, hand creams and lotions, lipstick, eye and face make-up, shaving cream and bubble bath soaps would have to be taken in fairly large amounts to cause problems. At worst there may be a little nausea and vomiting. Alimentary symptoms are more likely to follow consumption of thioglycollate-containing hair removers and bath salts.

Preparations containing ethanol (after-shave lotions, colognes, perfumes, mouth washes and hair lacquers) are amongst the most common toiletries ingested by children but serious intoxication

(p. 109) is unlikely. Occasionally, however, they are taken as cheap forms of alcohol by alcoholics.

The toluene and acetone contained in nail varnish and nail varnish removers are also potential causes of serious poisoning with CNS depression, hepatic and renal necrosis and cardiac dysrhythmias in extreme cases (p. 201 and 59), although features of this severity rarely occur after accidental poisoning in childhood.

Acute pulmonary oedema has been described in children after inhalation of large quantities of talc-containing powders and a few deaths have resulted.

Treatment

Unless there is good evidence that a large quantity of a toilet or cosmetic preparation has been ingested there is little merit in trying to empty the stomach. Even symptomatic treatment is unlikely to be required. In rare patients in whom consciousness is impaired or renal or hepatic damage has occurred treatment is supportive and conventional.

References

Lovejoy FH, Flowers J, McGuigan M. The epidemiology of poisoning from household products. *Vet Hum Toxicol* 1979; **21**: Suppl 33–34.

Lovejoy FH, Gouveia W, Edlin AI. Childhood poisoning with toilet and cosmetic articles. *Paediatrician* 1977; **6**: 226–243.

VERAPAMIL

General considerations

Verapamil is widely used in the treatment of angina of effort and supraventricular dysrhythmias. It depresses the sinoatrial and atrioventricular nodes probably by inhibiting the slow inflow of calcium ions during the plateau phase of the cardiac action potential. It also causes vasodilatation and inhibits insulin release.

Acute overdosage with verapamil is very uncommon but may be fatal. Verapamil is rapidly absorbed from the gastrointestinal tract and is extensively metabolised in the liver.

Features

The features of poisoning are normally apparent within 4 hours. Mental confusion and nausea have been reported. There is usually a marked bradycardia which may be sinus or nodal in origin, profound hypotension with cold, cyanosed extremities. Metabolic acidosis and hyperglycaemia may be present.

The electrocardiogram may show A-V block or A-V dissociation.

Treatment

The stomach should be emptied if the tablets have been ingested within 4 hours. Experience with verapamil poisoning is extremely limited and its definitive treatment remains uncertain. Atropine may reverse the bradycardia and improve A-V conduction. Calcium gluconate (10–20 ml of a 10% solution intravenously over 5–10 minutes) returned nodal rhythm to sinus rhythm in one case but was ineffective in others. Beta-adrenergic agonists are best avoided if the patient has a history of angina or dysrhythmias. Cardiac pacing may be necessary.

References

Da Silva OA, De Melo RA, Filho JPJ. Verapamil acute self-poisoning. *Clin Toxicol* 1979; **14**: 361–367.

de Faire U, Lundman T. Attempted suicide with verapamil. *Eur J Cardiol* 1977; **6**: 195–198.

Gelbke HP, Schlicht HJ, Schmidt G. Fatal poisoning with verapamil. *Arch Toxicol* 1977; **37**: 89–94.

Perkins CM. Serious verapamil poisoning: treatment with intravenous calcium gluconate. *Br Med J* 1978; **2**: 1127.

VILOXAZINE

General considerations

Viloxazine is a bicyclic antidepressant which is chemically unrelated to other antidepressants. It is well absorbed and almost completely metabolised. Less than 80 per cent of the circulating drug is bound to plasma proteins.

Features

There is very little information on the effects of acute overdosage with viloxazine. Drowsiness progressing to coma may occur with a slight rise in pulse rate and mild hypotension. Serious anticholinergic features have not been noted. One patient is reported to have died after a large overdose but details have not been published.

Treatment

It is probably unnecessary to empty the stomach unless more than 30 tablets (1.5 g) have been taken by an adult. Supportive measures should be instituted as indicated by the patient's clinical state.

Prognosis

Coma does not last longer than about 24 hours and recovery is usually complete within 36 hours.

Reference

Brosnan RD, Busby AM, Holland RPC. Cases of overdosage with viloxazine hydrochloride. *J Int Med Res* 1976; **4**:83–85.

WARFARIN

General considerations

Warfarin is a widely used anticoagulant which competes with vitamin K thereby blocking hepatic synthesis of factors II, VII, IX and X. It is also the active ingredient of some rodenticides but is present in such small quantities that large amounts would have to be eaten by a human before serious poisoning developed. Accidental and intentional acute poisoning are much less common than therapeutic overdosage.

Features

Spontaneous bleeding is the only important consequence of acute warfarin poisoning and usually occurs from the nose, gums and gastrointestinal and urinary tracts. Less commonly there may be haemorrhage into the skin and brain. However, even in overdosage, warfarin takes 24–60 hours to exert its maximum anticoagulant effect and most patients will present, asymptomatic, long before haemorrhage is likely.

Plasma warfarin concentrations

Plasma warfarin concentrations of up to 30 mg/l have been reported after deliberate self-poisoning and decay with a half-life of 24–72 hours. The usual therapeutic range for plasma warfarin concentrations is 1–3 mg/l.

Treatment

Individual susceptibility to warfarin varies considerably and it is recommended that the stomach should be emptied if more than 10 mg or twice the usual maintenance dose has been taken.

Treatment thereafter depends on whether or not the patient is on long-term anticoagulants, rapid reversal of which could be life-threatening (e.g. patients with prosthetic heart valves).

Patients not on anticoagulants should be given vitamin K_1 (10 mg intramuscularly daily) but if bleeding has already occurred fresh frozen plasma will be necessary for immediate control since vitamin K_1 will require about 24 hours to be effective.

Intravenous infusion of fresh frozen plasma is also the treatment of choice when it is undesirable to completely reverse the anticoagulant effect of warfarin. If possible the prothrombin time ratio should be kept below 3.0. It is essential to keep the patient under surveillance for several days because of the long plasma half-life of the drug. Warfarin should be restarted when fresh frozen plasma is no longer required and the prothrombin ratio is just slightly greater than the optimum for treatment.

WATER HEMLOCK

General considerations

Water hemlock is the common name given to the highly poisonous plants of the *Cicuta* genus of the Umbelliferae family. Poisoning usually results from ingestion of the roots in mistake for parsnips and as little as one rhizome may be fatal for an adult. *C. virosa*, the subspecies usually involved in poisoning episodes in Europe, contains oenanthotoxin whereas the problem North American species are *C. maculata* and *C. douglasii* which contain cicutoxin, an isomer of oenanthotoxin. Both toxins are unsaturated, 17-carbon, aliphatic alcohols.

Features

Symptoms commonly start within one hour of ingestion with malaise, nausea, hypersalivation, vomiting and abdominal cramps. The patient may be aware of palpitations but the most dramatic features of poisoning are extensor muscle spasms, opisthotonus and convulsions. The pupils are often dilated and cyanosis and pyrexia may be present. Both bradycardia and tachycardia have been described and although ECG changes may be found, they tend to be non-specific. Rare signs include parotid enlargement and flushing of the skin with subsequent desquamation.

There may be a polymorph leukocytosis and metabolic acidosis. High serum creatine phosphokinase and aspartate aminotransferase values occur commonly. Elevation of the former may be due to repeated convulsions but a toxic myositis has been postulated. Jaundice (in rare cases) and hypoprothrombinaemia suggest that hepatocellular damage may account for the raised aspartate aminotransferase.

Treatment

There is no specific treatment for water hemlock poisoning. The stomach should be emptied and convulsions controlled (p. 51). Other features should be treated symptomatically.

Prognosis

Water hemlock poisoning carries a much higher mortality than most plant poisonings but if convulsions and extensor spasms can be controlled the patient is usually considerably improved within 12 hours. There may be fever and muscle pain and weakness for a few days after recovery. Long-term mental impairment with EEG changes has been reported.

References

Carlton BE, Tufts E, Girard DE. Water hemlock poisoning complicated by rhabdomyolysis and renal failure. *Clin Toxicol* 1979; **14**:87–92.
Starreveld E, Hope CE. Cicutoxin poisoning (water hemlock). *Neurology* (*Minneap*) 1975; **25**:730–734.

YEW

General considerations

Various types of yew are commonly cultivated including *Taxus baccata* (the English yew), *T. canadensis* (the American yew) and *T. cuspidata* (the Japanese yew). The common name of the American yew, ground hemlock, is unfortunate since it is totally unrelated to the true hemlocks (*Conium* spp.).

All parts of the yew are poisonous including the berries which comprise a single seed all but enclosed in an attractive fleshy red cup. The toxic principle is an alkaloid, taxine, which is well absorbed, but the gastro-intestinal features of poisoning may be due to irritant oils. Poisoning with yew berries is uncommon.

Features

The usual features of poisoning include vomiting and abdominal pain with diarrhoea. Convulsions and impairment of consciousness may occur with respiratory depression. The lethal effects, however, are due to hypotension, bradycardia and depression of myocardial contractility and conductivity. Poisoning with yew berries is widely held to be extremely serious and some authors state that death is sudden and survival unlikely. In contrast, a recent French review reported that symptoms developed in only five out of thirty-three alleged ingestions.

Treatment

There is no specific treatment for this type of poisoning. The potential consequences are so serious that it would seem wise to empty the stomach if more than two or three berries have been ingested within 4 hours. Problems should then be dealt with as they arise.

Poisons information services

Eire

Dublin	Poisons Information Centre Jervis Street Hospital	0001–745588

England

Leeds	Leeds General Infirmary	0532–30715
London	National Poisons Information Service Guy's Hospital	01–407–7600

Northern Ireland

Belfast	Royal Victoria Hospital	0232–40503

Scotland

Edinburgh	Scottish Poisons Information Bureau Royal Infirmary	031–229–2477

Wales

Cardiff	Cardiff Royal Infirmary	0222–492233

Useful reference books

Collier WAL. *Imprex*, 7th ed. Cambridge: Imprex, 1978. (Index of imprints used on tablets and capsules.)

Duncan C. *MIMS Colour Index*. London; Medical Publications Ltd, 1981. (For tablet and capsule identification.)

Gosselin RE, Hodge HC, Smith RP, Gleason MN. *Clinical Toxicology of Commercial Products*, 4th ed. Baltimore: William & Wilkins, 1976.

Martindale's Extra Pharmacopoeia, 27th ed. London: The Pharmaceutical Press, 1977.

North P. *Poisonous Plants*. London: Blandford Press, 1967.

Vale JA, Meredith TJ. *Poisoning, diagnosis and treatment*. London: Update Publications, 1981.

Some proprietary preparations and their constituents

The constituents refer to tablets and capsules unless otherwise stated. Slow release formulations are denoted by asterisks.

Proprietary name	Constituents
Abstem	Calcium carbimide 50 mg
Actidil	Triprolidine 2.5 mg
Actifed	Triprolidine 2.5 mg, pseudoephedrine 60 mg
Adalat	Nifedipine 10 mg
Aldomet	Methyldopa 125, 250, 500 mg
Allegron	Nortriptyline 10, 25 mg
Alupent	Orciprenaline 10 mg
syrup	Orciprenaline 10 mg in 5 ml
Amesec	Aminophylline 150 mg, ephedrine 25 mg, amylobarbitone 25 mg
Amytal	Amylobarbitone 15, 30, 50, 100, 200 mg
Anafranil	Clomipramine 10, 25, 50 mg
Angiers Junior Aspirin	Acetylsalicylic acid 81 mg
Antabuse	Disulfiram 200 mg
Anthisan	Mepyramine maleate 50, 100 mg
elixir	Mepyramine maleate 25 mg in 5 ml
Apisate	Diethylpropion 75 mg and B vitamins
Artane	Benzhexol 2, 5 mg
*sustets	Benzhexol 5 mg
Askit	Acetylsalicylic acid 260 mg, aloxiprin 120 mg, caffeine 20 mg
powders	Acetylsalicylic acid 750 mg, aloxiprin 200 mg, caffeine 110 mg
Asmapax	Ephedrine 50 mg, theophylline 65 mg, bromvaletone 200 mg
Aspro	Acetylsalicylic acid 324 mg
clear	Acetylsalicylic acid 300 mg
effervescent	Acetylsalicylic acid 300 mg
Atarax	Hydroxyzine 10, 15 mg

Ativan	Lorazepam 1, 2.5 mg
Aventyl	Nortriptyline 10, 25 mg
Avloclor	Chloroquine 250 mg
Avomine	Promethazine 25 mg
Beechams	Acetylsalicylic acid 270 mg, salicylamide 25 mg, caffeine 10 mg
powders	Acetylsalicylic acid 540 mg, salicylamide 50 mg, caffeine 10 mg
Belladenal	Belladonna alkaloids 0.25 mg, phenobarbitone 50 mg
*retard	Belladonna alkaloids 0.25 mg, phenobarbitone 50 mg
Bellergal	Belladonna alkaloids 0.1 mg, ergotamine 0.3 mg, phenobarbitone 20 mg
*retard	Belladonna alkaloids 0.2 mg, ergotamine 0.6 mg, phenobarbitone 40 mg
Benadryl	Diphenhydramine 25 mg
Benoral	Benorylate 750 mg
suspension	Benorylate 4 g in 10 ml
Benylin Expectorant	Diphenhydramine 14 mg, ammonium chloride 135 mg in 5 ml
Benylin Paediatric	Diphenhydramine 7 mg in 5 ml
Beta-Cardone	Sotalol 40, 80, 200 mg
Betaloc	Metoprolol 50, 100 mg
*Betaloc-SA	Metoprolol 200 mg
Bolvidon	Mianserin 10, 20, 30 mg
Brufen	Ibuprofen 200 mg
400	Ibuprofen 400 mg
Buscopan	Hyoscine butylbromide 10 mg
Butazolidin	Phenylbutazone 100, 200 mg
Cafergot	Ergotamine 1 mg, caffeine 100 mg
Camcolit 250	Lithium carbonate 250 mg
400	Lithium carbonate 400 mg
Carbrital	Pentobarbitone sodium 97.5 mg, carbromal 260 mg
Carisoma	Carisoprodol 125, 350 mg
Carisoma Compound	Carisoprodol 175 mg, paracetamol 350 mg, caffeine 32 mg
Catapres	Clonidine 0.1, 0.3 mg
Cedilanid	Lanatoside C 0.25 mg
Centyl-K	Bendrofluazide 2.5 mg, potassium 7.7 mmol
Cetiprin	Emepronium 100, 200 mg
Choledyl	Choline theophyllinate 100, 200 mg
Clinitest reagent	Sodium hydroxide
Codis	Acetylsalicylic acid 500 mg, codeine phosphate 8 mg
Cogentin	Benztropine 2 mg

Colofac	Mebeverine 135 mg
Concordin	Protriptyline 5, 10 mg
Cordilox	Verapamil 40, 80 mg
Cosalgesic	Dextropropoxyphene 32.5 mg, paracetamol 325 mg
Cyclimorph 10	Morphine 10 mg, cyclizine 50 mg in 1 ml ampoule
Dalmane	Flurazepam 15, 30 mg
Duraprim	Pyrimethamine 25 mg
*Debendox	Dicyclomine 10 mg, doxylamine 10 mg, pyridoxine 10 mg
Declinax	Debrisoquine 10, 20 mg
Depixol	Flupenthixol 20 mg in 1 ml ampoule
*Depronal SA	Dextropropoxyphene 150 mg
Dexedrine	Dexamphetamine 5 mg
DF 118	Dihydrocodeine 30 mg
elixir	Dihydrocodeine 10 mg in 5 ml
Diabinese	Chlorpropamide 100, 250 mg
Dibotin	Phenformin 25 mg
Diconal	Dipipanone 10 mg, cyclizine 30 mg
Digitaline Nativelle	Digitoxin 0.1 mg
Dindevan	Phenindione 10, 25, 50 mg
Disipal	Orphenadrine 50 mg
Disprin	Acetylsalicylic acid 300 mg, calcium carbonate 90 mg, citric acid 30 mg
junior	Acetylsalicylic acid 81 mg, calcium carbonate 90 mg, citric acid 8 mg
Distalgesic	Dextropropoxyphene 32.5 mg, paracetamol 325 mg
Dixarit	Clonidine 25 µg
Do Do	Ephedrine 22 mg, theophylline 30 mg, caffeine 30 mg, salicylamide 30 mg, lobeline 100 µg
Dolasan	Dextropropoxyphene 100 mg, aspirin 325 mg
Dolobid	Diflunisal 250 mg
Doloxene	Dextropropoxyphene 65 mg
Doloxene Compound	Dextropropoxyphene 65 mg, acetylsalicylic acid 375 mg, caffeine 30 mg
Doriden	Glutethimide 250 mg
Drinamyl	Dexamphetamine sulphate 5 mg, amylobarbitone 32 mg
*Duromine	Phentermine 15, 30 mg
Durophet	Amphetamine and dexamphetamine in equal parts, 7.5, 12.5, 20 mg
Durophet M	Amphetamine and dexamphetamine in equal parts, 12.5, 20 mg, methaqualone 40 mg
Eltroxin	Thyroxine 50, 100 µg

Epanutin	Phenytoin 25, 50, 100 mg
suspension	Phenytoin 30 mg in 5 ml
Epilim	Sodium valproate 200, 500 mg
Equagesic	Ethoheptazine 75 mg, meprobamate 150 mg, aspirin 250 mg, calcium carbonate 75 mg
Equanil	Meprobamate 200, 400 mg
Esbatal	Bethanidine 10, 50 mg
Etophylate	Acepifylline 250 mg
Euhypnos	Temazepam 10 mg
forte	Temazepam 20 mg
Febrilix Elixir	Paracetamol 120 mg in 5 ml
Fefol Spansule	Ferrous sulphate 150 mg, folic acid 0.5 mg
Feminax	Paracetamol 250 mg, salicylamide 250 mg, codeine phosphate 10 mg, caffeine 10 mg, hyoscine 100 µg
Fentazin	Perphenazine 2, 4, 8 mg
Feospan	Ferrous sulphate 150 mg
*Ferrograd C	Ferrous sulphate 325 mg, ascorbic acid 500 mg
*Ferro-Gradumet	Ferrous sulphate 325 mg
Fersamal	Ferrous fumarate (equivalent to 65 mg iron)
syrup	Ferrous fumarate 140 mg in 5 ml
Filon	Phenbutrazate 20 mg, phenmetrazine 20 mg
Fluanxol	Flupenthixol 0.5 mg
Fortagesic	Pentazocine 15 mg, paracetamol 500 mg
Fortral	Pentazocine 25, 50 mg
Franol	Ephedrine 11 mg, theophylline 120 mg, phenobarbitone 8 mg
Franol Plus	Ephedrine 15 mg, theophylline 120 mg, thenyldiamine 10 mg, phenobarbitone 8 mg
Frisium	Clobazam 10 mg
Glibenese	Glipizide 5 mg
Glucophage	Metformin 500, 850 mg
Halcion	Triazolam 0.125, 0.25 mg
Haliborange	Vitamin A 750 µg, vitamin D 5 µg, ascorbic acid 25 mg
Hedex	Paracetamol 500 mg
Hedex Seltzer	Paracetamol 1 g, caffeine 60 mg, sodium bicarbonate 1.54 g, citric acid 1.24 g
Heminevrin	Chlormethiazole edisylate 500 mg
capsules	Chlormethiazole 192 mg in arachis oil
syrup	Chlormethiazole edisylate 250 mg in 5 ml
*Histryl	Diphenylpyraline 5 mg
Hypon	Acetylsalicylic acid 325 mg, caffeine 10 mg, codeine 5 mg
Imodium	Loperamide 2 mg

Inderal	Propranolol 40, 80, 160 mg
Indocid	Indomethacin 25, 50 mg
Integrin	Oxypertine 10 mg
Kemadrin	Procyclidine 5 mg
Kinidin	Quinidine 250 mg
Lanoxin	Digoxin 0.125, 0.25 mg
PG	Digoxin 62.5 µg
Largactil	Chlorpromazine 25, 50, 100 mg
Lemsip	Paracetamol 650 mg, phenylephrine 5 mg, ascorbic acid 10 mg, sodium citrate 500 mg per sachet
Lemsip Junior	Paracetamol 217 mg, phenylephrine 1.7 mg, ascorbic acid 3.3 mg, sodium citrate 167 mg per sachet
*Lentizol	Amitriptyline 25, 50 mg
Leo K	Potassium chloride 600 mg (potassium 8 mmol)
Libraxin	Chlordiazepoxide 5 mg, clidinium bromide 2.5 mg
Librium	Chlordiazepoxide 5, 10, 25 mg
Limbitrol	Amitriptyline 25 mg, chlordiazepoxide 10 mg
Lioresal	Baclofen 10 mg
Lobak	Chlormezanone 100 mg, paracetamol 450 mg
Lomotil	Diphenoxylate 2.5 mg, atropine 0.025 mg
Lopresor	Metoprolol 50, 100 mg
Ludiomil	Maprotiline 10, 25, 50, 75, 150 mg
Luminal	Phenobarbitone 15, 30, 60 mg
Mandrax	Methaqualone 250 mg, diphenhydramine 25 mg
Marevan	Warfarin 1, 3, 5, 10 mg
Marplan	Isocarboxazid 10 mg
Marsilid	Iproniazid 25, 50 mg
Maxolon	Metoclopramide 10 mg
Medomin	Heptabarbitone 200 mg
Melleril	Thioridazine 10, 25, 50, 100 mg
Merbentyl	Dicyclomine 10 mg
Merital	Nomifensine 25, 50 mg
Mexitil	Mexiletine 50, 200 mg
Migraleve (pink)	Buclizine 6.25 mg, paracetamol 500 mg, codeine 8 mg, dioctylsodium sulphosuccinate 10 mg
yellow	Paracetamol 500 mg, codeine 8 mg, dioctylsodium sulphosuccinate 20 mg
Migril	Ergotamine 2 mg, cyclizine 50 mg, caffeine 100 mg
Miltown	Meprobamate 200, 400 mg
Modecate	Fluphenazine 25 mg per ml
Moditen	Fluphenazine 1, 2.5, 5 mg
elixir	Fluphenazine 0.5 mg in 1 ml

Mogadon	Nitrazepam 5 mg
Molipaxin	Trazodone 50, 100 mg
Motipress	Fluphenazine 1.5 mg, nortriptyline 30 mg
Motival	Fluphenazine 0.5 mg, nortriptyline 10 mg
Myambutol	Ethambutol 100, 400 mg
Mysoline	Primidone 250 mg
Napsalgesic	Dextropropoxyphene 50 mg, acetylsalicylic acid 500 mg
Narcan	Naloxone 0.4 mg in 1 ml ampoule
Nardil	Phenelzine 15 mg
Narphen	Phenazocine 5 mg
Navidrex-K	Cyclopenthiazide 0.25 mg, potassium chloride 600 mg (8 mmol potassium)
Nembutal	Pentobarbitone 50, 100 mg
*Neo-Naclex-K	Bendrofluazide 2.5 mg, potassium chloride 630 mg (8.4 mmol potassium)
Night Nurse	Promethazine 20 mg, pholcodine 10 mg, paracetamol 500 mg, alcohol 3.08 ml in 20 ml syrup
Nivaquine	Chloroquine 200 mg
Nobrium	Medazepam 5, 10 mg
Noctec	Chloral hydrate 500 mg
Noludar	Methyprylone 200 mg
Norgesic	Orphenadrine 35 mg, paracetamol 450 mg
Normison	Temazepam 10, 20 mg
Norpace	Disopyramide 150 mg
Norval	Mianserin 10, 20, 30 mg
Nu-Seals Aspirin	Acetylsalicylic acid 300, 600 mg
Oblivon	Methylpentynol 250 mg
Omnopon	Papaveretum 10 mg
Optimax	l-Tryptophan 500 mg, pyridoxine 5 mg, ascorbic acid 10 mg
Orap	Pimozide 2, 4 mg
Ospolot	Sulthiame 50, 200 mg
Palfium	Dextromoramide 5, 10 mg
Panadeine Co	Paracetamol 500 mg, codeine 8 mg
Panadol	Paracetamol 500 mg
Panasorb	Paracetamol 500 mg
Paracodol	Paracetamol 500 mg, codeine 8 mg
Paragesic	Paracetamol 500 mg, pseudoephedrine 20 mg, caffeine 10 mg
Parahypon	Paracetamol 500 mg, caffeine 10 mg, codeine 5 mg
Paramax	Paracetamol 500 mg, metoclopramide 5 mg
Paramol 118	Paracetamol 500 mg, dihydrocodeine 10 mg
Para-Seltzer	Paracetamol 500 mg, caffeine 20 mg

Parnate	Tranylcypromine 10 mg
Parstelin	Tranylcypromine 10 mg, trifluoperazine 1 mg
Paynocil	Acetylsalicylic acid 600 mg, aminoacetic acid 300 mg
Persomnia	Salicylamide 375 mg, paracetamol 150 mg
Pertofran	Desipramine 25 mg
Phenergan	Promethazine 10, 25 mg
Phensic	Acetylsalicylic acid 325 mg, caffeine 50 mg
*Phyllocontin	Aminophylline 225 mg
Physeptone	Methadone 5 mg
linctus	Methadone 2 mg in 5 ml
Piriton	Chlorpheniramine 4 mg
Plaquenil	Hydroxychloroquine 200 mg
Ponderax	Fenfluramine 20, 40 mg
*Ponderax PA	Fenfluramine 60 mg
Ponstan	Mefenamic acid 250 mg
forte	Mefenamic acid 500 mg
Potter's Asthma Remedy	Stramonium leaves
Priadel	Lithium carbonate 400 mg
*Pro-Actidil	Triprolidine 10 mg
Pro-Banthine	Propantheline 15 mg
Pronestyl	Procainamide 250 mg
Pro-Plus	Caffeine 50 mg
Prothiaden	Dothiepin 25, 75 mg
Quellada	Gamma-benzene hexachloride 1% lotion
Quick Kwells	Hyoscine 300 µg
Reactivan	Fencamfamin 10 mg and B vitamins
Remnos	Nitrazepam 5, 10 mg
Rinurel	Paracetamol 300 mg, phenylpropanolamine 25 mg, phenyltoloxamine 22 mg
Ritalin	Methylphenidate 10 mg
Rivotril	Clonazepam 0.5, 2 mg
Rythmodan	Disopyramide 100, 150 mg
Safapryn	Acetylsalicylic acid 300 mg, paracetamol 250 mg
Safapryn-Co	Acetylsalicylic acid 300 mg, paracetamol 250 mg, codeine 8 mg
Sanomigran	Pizotifen 0.5 mg
Saroten	Amitriptyline 10, 25 mg
Seconal	Quinalbarbitone 50, 100 mg
Sectral	Acebutal 100, 200 mg
Serenace	Haloperidol 0.5 mg
Serenid-D	Oxazepam 10, 15 mg
forte	Oxazepam 30 mg
Sinequan	Doxepin 10, 25 mg
*Slow-Trasicor	Oxprenolol 160 mg

Sodium Amytal	Amylobarbitone sodium 60, 200 mg
Solpadeine	Paracetamol 500 mg, codeine phosphate 8 mg, caffeine 30 mg
Solprin	Acetylsalicylic acid 300 mg
Somnased	Nitrazepem 5 mg
Sonalgin	Butobarbitone 60 mg, codeine 10 mg, paracetamol 375 mg
Soneryl	Butobarbitone 100 mg
Sotacor	Sotalol 80, 160 mg
Sparine	Promazine 25, 50, 100 mg
Stelazine	Trifluoperazine 1, 2, 5, 10, 15 mg
Stemetil	Prochlorperazine 5, 25 mg
Sudafed	Pseudoephedrine 60 mg
Surmontil	Trimipramine 10, 25, 50 mg
Tacitin	Benzoctamine 10 mg
Tagamet	Cimetidine 200 mg
Tedral	Theophylline 120 mg, ephedrine 24 mg, phenobarbitone 8 mg
Tegretol	Carbamazepine 100, 200 mg
Temgesic	Buprenorphine 0.3 mg per ml
Tenormin	Atenolol 100 mg
Tenuate	Diethylpropion 25 mg
*Tenuate dospan	Diethylpropion 75 mg
Tofranil	Imipramine 10, 25 mg
Torecan	Thiethylperazine 10 mg
Trancopal	Chlormezanone 200 mg
Trandate	Labetalol 100, 200, 400 mg
Tranxene	Chlorazepate 15 mg
Trasicor	Oxprenolol 20, 40, 80, 160 mg
Tricloryl	Triclofos sodium 500 mg
Triogesic	Phenylpropanolamine 12.5 mg, paracetamol 500 mg
Triptafen DA	Amitriptyline 25 mg, perphenazine 2 mg
Tryptizol	Amitriptyline 10, 25, 50, 75 mg
Tuinal	Quinalbarbitone and amylobarbitone in equal parts 100, 200 mg
Valium	Diazepam 2, 5, 10 mg
Vallergan	Trimeprazine 10 mg
Veganin	Acetylsalicylic acid 250 mg, paracetamol 250 mg, codeine 10 mg
Ventolin	Salbutamol 2, 4 mg
Vivalan	Viloxazine 50 mg

Common names used by addicts

A	amphetamine	Happy dust	cocaine
Acid	LSD	Hard stuff	morphine
Amphet	amphetamine	Harry	heroin
Angel dust	phencyclidine	Hash	cannabis resin
Barbs	barbiturate	Hash oil	cannabis oil
Bernice	cocaine	Hog	phencyclidine
Bhang	cannabis	Horse	heroin
Blues	amphetamine	Ice	cocaine
Boy	heroin	Joint	cannabis
Brown sugar	heroin	Joy powder	heroin
Bush	cannabis	Junk	heroin
C	cocaine	Leaf	cocaine
Charlie	cocaine	M	morphine
Chinese	heroin	Marijuana	cannabis
Chinese rock	heroin	Mandies	methaqualone
Coke	cocaine	Mary Jane	cannabis
Crystal	phencyclidine	Miss Emma	morphine
Dexies	dexamphetamine	Monkey	morphine
Dike	dipipanone	Morf	morphine
Doll	methadone	Morpho	morphine
Dollies	methadone	Nembies	pentobarbitone
Dome dots	LSD	Paki	cannabis
Domes	LSD	Paradise	cocaine
Dope	cannabis	PCP	phencyclidine
Dots	LSD	PeaCe pill	phencyclidine
Downers	barbiturates	Pot	cannabis
DP (Durban		Reefer	cannabis
poison)	cannabis	Resin	cannabis resin
Dreamer	morphine	Rock	heroin
Dynamite	cocaine	Rock'n roll	heroin
Elephant	heroin	Seccies	quinalbarbitone
Flake	cocaine	Shit	cannabis
Ganja	cannabis	Smack	heroin
Grass	cannabis	Smoke	cannabis
H	heroin	Snow	cocaine

Sodies	sodium amylobarbitine	Thai sticks	cannabis
Speed	amphetamine and other stimulants	Thing	heroin
		Uppers	amphetamine
		Wake ups	amphetamine
Speedball	cocaine with heroin	Weed	cannabis
Split	cannabis	White	
Stuff	heroin	elephant	heroin
Sulph	amphetamine	White stuff	heroin
Tea	cannabis		

Conversion factors for drug concentrations

To convert:

Drug	Molar Units to	Mass Units	Multiply by
Amitriptyline (base)	μmol/l	μg/l	277.4
Barbiturates			
amylobarbitone	μmol/l	mg/l	0.226
butobarbitone	μmol/l	mg/l	0.212
cyclobarbitone	μmol/l	mg/l	0.236
pentobarbitone	μmol/l	mg/l	0.226
phenobarbitone	μmol/l	mg/l	0.232
quinalbarbitone	μmol/l	mg/l	0.238
Carbamazepine	μmol/l	mg/l	0.236
Chlormethiazole (base)	μmol/l	mg/l	0.1615
Digoxin	nmol/l	μg/l	0.781
Ethanol	mmol/l	mg/l	46.0
Glutethimide	μmol/l	mg/l	0.217
Imipramine (base)	μmol/l	μg/l	230.4
Iron	μmol/l	μg/l	55.85
Isopropanol	mmol/l	mg/l	60.1
Meprobamate	mmol/l	mg/l	218.3
Methanol	mmol/l	mg/l	32.0
Methaqualone	μmol/l	mg/l	0.25
Paracetamol	mmol/l	mg/l	151.2
Phenytoin	μmol/l	mg/l	0.252
Quinine	μmol/l	mg/l	0.325
Salicylate	mmol/l	mg/l	138.1
Theophylline	μmol/l	mg/l	0.13

Clearly molar units may be obtained by dividing mass units by the same factors.

Index

DATE DUE